Working with Communication and Swallowing Difficulties in Older Adults

This accessible resource offers valuable guidance for all student and practising speech and language therapists (SLTs) who are working with older people with communication and swallowing difficulties. Chapters provide up-to-date theory on age-related changes alongside practical strategies for clinicians to use in their daily work, from helping with mental capacity decisions to supporting older people with good palliative care.

Promoting a holistic approach for ageing well, this resource dispels myths that surround the ageing process while detailing the normal physiological and psychological effects of ageing on communication and swallowing, as well as diseases and conditions associated with older age, such as frailty.

Illustrated throughout with clinical case studies and helpful photocopiable resources to use in practice, this book is a key part of the toolkit for any speech and language therapist working with older adults.

Rebecca Allwood is a practising speech and language therapist specialising in older adults. She has been practising for over seventeen years and has worked in a variety of clinical settings with older adults who have communication and swallowing difficulties.

The *Working With* Series

The *Working With* series provides speech and language therapists with a range of 'go-to' resources, full of well-sourced, up-to-date information regarding specific disorders. Underpinned by robust theoretical foundations and supported by intervention options and exercises, every book ensures that the reader has access to the latest thinking regarding diagnosis, management and treatment options.

Written in a fully accessible style, each book bridges theory and practice and offers ready-to-use and well-rehearsed practical material, including guidance on interventions, management advice, and therapeutic resources for the client, parent or carer. The series is an invaluable resource for practitioners, whether speech and language therapy students, or more experienced clinicians.

Books in the series include:

Working with Children's Language, 2nd edition
Diana Williams
2022 / pb: 9780367467913

Working with Voice Disorders: Theory and Practice, 3rd edition
Stephanie Martin
2021 / pb: 9780863889462

Working with Communication and Swallowing Difficulties in Older Adults
Rebecca Allwood
2022 / pb: 9780367524784

Working with Solution Focused Brief Therapy in Healthcare Settings
Kidge Burns and Sarah Northcott
2022 / pb: 9780367435097

Working with Communication and Swallowing Difficulties in Older Adults

Rebecca Allwood

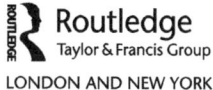

Routledge
Taylor & Francis Group

LONDON AND NEW YORK

Cover image: @Getty Images

First published 2022
by Routledge
4 Park Square, Milton Park, Abingdon, Oxon OX14 4RN

and by Routledge
605 Third Avenue, New York, NY 10158

Routledge is an imprint of the Taylor & Francis Group, an informa business

British Library Cataloguing-in-Publication Data
A catalogue record for this book is available from the British Library

Library of Congress Cataloging-in-Publication Data
A catalog record for this book has been requested

ISBN: 978-0-367-52480-7 (hbk)
ISBN: 978-0-367-52478-4 (pbk)
ISBN: 978-1-003-05809-0 (ebk)

DOI: 10.4324/9781003058090

Typeset in Interstate
by Apex CoVantage, LLC

Access the Companion Website: www.routledge.com/cw/speechmark

Contents

Acknowledgements

With huge gratitude to Dr Stephanie Martin for her continued guidance, support and wisdom throughout the process of writing this book. And to Professor Rowan Harwood, geriatrician, for giving his support and encouragement and for being an inspirational advocate of a multidisciplinary approach to healthcare for older people.

Thank you to my speech and language therapy colleagues for their support and willingness to engage in discussions related to the material in this book and to those colleagues who have read through and commented on chapters: Jane Stockwell, Tilly Archer, Tiffany Green and Siân Rajakaruna.

Grateful thanks to those who have offered their time and expertise: Emma Grace (pharmacist), Rachel Lyon (dietitian), Samantha Littlefair (lecturer in speech and language therapy) and Dr Anna Henderson (General Practitioner).

It is a true privilege to work as a speech and language therapist in the field of healthcare for older people. Thank you to my patients who have taught me so much over the years.

INTRODUCTION

Welcome to *Working with Communication and Swallowing Difficulties in Older Adults*. This is a go-to resource for speech and language therapy students and speech and language therapists starting work with older people. It will be of interest and benefit to wider health and social care professionals, as many of their older clients will experience communication and swallowing difficulties.

This resource delves into a number of topics related to communication and swallowing in older age, from the physiology of ageing and rehabilitation, working with an older client group, assessment and management of communication and swallowing in older people, decision making, and palliative care. There is discussion on current topics, including the impact of frailty and advanced care planning.

Clinical resources and practical tips are available throughout the book.

Whilst older adults have always represented a significant proportion of adult speech and language therapy caseloads, speech and language therapy within the field of healthcare for older people is becoming more distinct and viewed as its own expertise. It is a fulfilling, dynamic area to work in, requiring innovation, flexibility and problem solving skills to meet the communication and swallowing needs of our older population.

I hope that you will enjoy reading and using this resource, and that it will become a valuable part of your toolkit when working with older adults who have communication and swallowing difficulties.

DOI: 10.4324/9781003058090-1

AN OVERVIEW OF AGEING AND AN INTRODUCTION TO THIS RESOURCE

DOI: 10.4324/9781003058090-2

The context of ageing

The world's population of older people is increasing. The World Health Organisation (WHO) predicts nearly a doubling of the proportion of people in the world who are over 60 years of age from 12% in 2020 to 22% in 2050. This estimate means that by 2050, almost a quarter of the world's population will be over 60.

The age at which a person is referred to as being in older age varies but is usually cited as being 60 and over, or 65 and over. In healthcare terms, older age is usually considered to be anyone 65 or over. In recent years, there has been a trend towards living into much older age. In the UK, the number of centenarians increased by 11% in 2019 compared to the number in 2018 (Office for National Statistics, 2020). With older age being designated as 60 or 65, this means that many people will be living in older age for around 30 years or more, which is a significant proportion of their lives.

There are inevitable physiological changes within the body due to the process of ageing. However, the rate and severity of these changes vary from person to person and interact with social and psychological factors, making one person's experience of being in older age very different from that of another.

Advances in medical treatments and improved living conditions can be hailed as contributors to people living into much older age. However, from a social, health and economic point of view, the infrastructure to support people to live with reasonable quality of life in much older age is limited in many countries. This is partially due to the pace of increase in the ageing population, which grew more rapidly in recent years (WHO, 2018). The recent COVID-19 pandemic shone a spotlight on the vulnerability of some older adults. Old age was an independent risk factor of serious illness and death from the virus. Nursing homes became hotspots for virus transmission and huge numbers of older people were shielded in their homes for months without real human contact.

This introductory chapter will address the wider context of the impact of ageing and healthcare for older people and begin to discuss how communication and swallowing are affected by the ageing process. Towards the end of the chapter is a section highlighting who will benefit from reading the book and how to use it as a clinical resource.

The impact of ageing

For many older adults, ageing is a positive experience. There is the wisdom gained from being able to reflect on many years of life. It can bring a freedom from the years of work and instigate a time for travelling and focusing on other interests. Relationships can grow, and there can be opportunities to meet new people. Family dynamics may also change positively with the arrival of grandchildren or great-grandchildren. Some older people enjoy maintaining paid or volunteer work.

On the other side of the picture, these benefits of older age are not available to all. Some people work into older age without a choice just so that they can afford to live. Families may live far apart from each other, or older people may be required to leave their home and move closer to family members. It is not uncommon for older people to take on caring duties for their own partners in declining health or to look after grandchildren.

One area that has gained increasing attention over recent years has been the level of loneliness amongst older people. Age UK (2018) reported that 1 in 12 older people in the UK report that they often feel lonely. Moving house, losing partners or friends and being in ill health are all factors that can increase the feelings of loneliness in old age.

Loneliness and social isolation are correlated with poor health outcomes. A systematic review and meta-analysis by Valtorta et al. (2016) found inadequate social relationships were associated with an increased risk of coronary heart disease and stroke.

Fortunately, the increased recognition of loneliness in later life has led to the development of charities and groups aiming to alleviate this. In the UK, there are various charities with the sole focus of support for older people, including educational and interest groups, face-to-face groups, and befriending and telephone support services.

The recent COVID-19 pandemic has been a setback for older people in terms of social isolation and feelings of being alone. The restrictions on face-to-face visiting in family or care homes, and the cancellation of many activities and groups have led to a significant increase in feelings of isolation, which could lead to long-term negative effects on health and wellbeing (Wu, 2020).

Health needs increase with ageing, and there is a distinction to be made between living in older age and living in older age with quality of life. Public Health England report that life expectancy in the UK has risen more quickly than healthy life expectancy, which means the years spent living in poor health has also increased (PHE, 2018). Comorbidities and long-term health conditions, such as diabetes, hypertension, arthritis and frailty, are more prevalent in older age, and increasing age is associated with the risk of developing illnesses, such as cancer, heart disease and stroke. Kingston et al. (2018) found over half of older people live with at least two chronic conditions and that this multimorbidity increases likelihood of consequences, such as hospital admission and readmission, increased dependency on care and mortality.

Of course, quality of life is subjective, and many older people adapt their lifestyles and adjust to changes. For other people, ill health and decline in function will bring a significant sense of loss and low mood, thereby increasing the risk of mental illness. It is estimated that around 40% of older people registered at GP practices have mental ill health, rising to around 60% in care homes (Social Care Institute for Excellence, 2006).

In some cultures, old age is revered, and older generations are respected for their wisdom and experience. In other cultures, there is an underlying message of preferred youthfulness, and advertisements for anti-ageing skin and hair products endorse this view. Similarly, spoken and written language can also discriminate against people in older age through the use of terms for people in older age that would be classed as pejorative.

With the negative aspects of ageing aside, older adults make up a large portion of our population, and the younger population would not be alive without them. Ageing with poor health is not inevitable, and it pays on a human, social and economic level to put efforts into keeping people healthy and with quality of life for as long as possible.

Communication and swallowing impairments in older age

This book is dedicated to the effects of communication and swallowing impairments in later life. Although communication and swallowing appear to be two different categories, they are linked in that both are vital for sustaining life and both contribute to quality of life. Both are subject to changes with the natural ageing process, and many of the diseases that are more prevalent in older age will have symptoms related to both communication and swallowing. The two are drawn together in the profession of speech and language therapy. Speech and language therapists (SLTs) are highly trained in the assessment and management of both communication and swallowing impairments.

The ability to communicate effectively is a fundamental aspect of life. At a basic level, we communicate to get our needs met; for example, communicating thirst or hunger or the need for emotional support. We also enjoy communicating for the purpose of social interaction and building relationships. As we age, aspects of communication change, and older people might not be able to communicate with the same ease as they did when they were younger. There are various physiological ways in which communication can be affected during the ageing process. For example, there are changes to hearing and sight, reduced processing speed and increased difficulty with word retrieval. These interact with lifestyle changes, such as retirement, moving into care homes or reduced mobility. Hearing loss in older people can lead to a lower quality of social interaction, which in turn might lead to reduced communication skills. Hearing impairment is directly associated with social isolation (Shukla et al., 2020). Research into hearing loss and dementia indicated a link with increasing severity of hearing loss and increased likelihood of developing dementia (Lin et al., 2011).

The process of eating, drinking and swallowing is essential to maintain life. The process spans many aspects of life, from physical and physiological to social, psychological and cultural. Lifestyle and physiological changes associated with ageing can make eating, drinking and swallowing in older age a different experience to that of a younger person. There are more common adaptations in later life, such as denture wearing occurring alongside less noticeable but significant changes, such as muscle weakness affecting the ability to chew and swallow effectively.

How ageing affects communication and swallowing will be discussed in detail in later chapters. Communication and swallowing feature prominently in other aspects of ageing, such as decision making about care, and in palliative and end of life care, which will also be discussed further on in the book.

The older population in healthcare

It may appear ageist or even discriminatory to talk about older people in a class of their own or to treat them as a special subset of patient group rather than as a general adult client group. The medical field have only in the last century started to define older people as a separate patient group. Interest in the healthcare of older people started to rise in the 1930s and 1940s. 'Care of the aged' was then included within the establishment of the National Health Service in 1948 (Morley, 2004), and the British Geriatrics Society was formed in 1947 (BGS, 2020).

Although granted that there is heterogeneity of ageing effects on an individual, ageing does indeed affect everybody. This will lead to unique needs for an older population compared with younger adults, and this will need to be accounted for by clinicians. Many illnesses and diseases are more prevalent in older age as a result of an ageing immune system.

Table 1.1 Common members of a multidisciplinary team specialising in healthcare for older people

The multidisciplinary team
General practitioner (GP)
Consultant specialising in older person's care (geriatrician)
Psychiatrist specialising in older person's care
Community psychiatric nurse / mental health nurse
Psychologist
District nurse
Occupational therapist
Speech and language therapist
Physiotherapist
Dietitian
Social worker
Care workers

Symptoms of these will be experienced against the background of age-related changes, which means that the disease will have different effects on older physiology to that of younger physiology.

The older body metabolises medication differently (Le Couteur et al., 2012), which needs special consideration in terms of side effects and effectiveness (see Chapter 3 for more detail). Age increases the likelihood of experiencing more vague and subtle symptoms of illness, which can lead to misdiagnosis and poor clinical outcomes if these have not been thoroughly investigated with special attention to the influence of age-related change (Hofman et al., 2017). An infection in older age is much more likely to trigger delirium or confusion than in a younger population.

Older people benefit when their health and social needs are provided for by a multidisciplinary team. The members of this team need to be experts in their particular area of health or social care and also experts in their knowledge of how the ageing process can affect an individual. Table 1.1 lists some of the common members of a multidisciplinary team involved in an older person's care.

How to use this book as a clinical resource

This book is primarily aimed at SLT students and newly qualified SLTs embarking on a clinical role working with older adults. It would also benefit more experienced SLTs entering a new clinical field working with older people or pre-reading for a clinical placement.

Whilst SLT students and SLTs are the most obvious clinical profession to benefit from this book as they specifically work with communication and swallowing impairment, this book would also be useful for any clinician in the wider multidisciplinary team working with older adults. Older people may first present to another professional, such as their local doctor or a dietitian, with complaints about communication or swallowing symptoms. These professionals need to have some awareness of these symptoms in older people in order to assist them in identifying normal age-related communication and swallowing problems, and what symptoms might necessitate referral to an SLT service and/or further investigation of a potential medical diagnosis. It will also help this professional to be able to provide interim advice and strategies whilst the person awaits an appointment with a speech and language therapist.

There is nothing that can truly take the place of practise-based learning in real-life situations. In order to gain true experience, students or clinicians need to learn by working alongside specialist colleagues and practising their skills on clients in real clinical encounters. Many speech and language therapy university courses include general observation placements with older people in care homes during the early stages of the course to enable students to learn about the typical changes of older age. This book is designed to be a practical resource to accompany a student or clinician in their clinical development and understanding of working with older people with communication and swallowing difficulties.

This resource provides a broad range of important topics to have knowledge of when working with older people who have communication and/or swallowing problems, and spans the process of normal ageing, pathological ageing and other features of ageing, such as decision making and palliative care. The objective is to give a detailed overview of each topic so that the reader can use it as a reference and a practical tool but can select some of the topics to study in more detail if there is a particular interest.

Throughout, there are examples of clinical resources that clinicians can use in their practise. These include case history proformas, symptom checklists, and information and exercise sheets. There are case studies in several of the chapters, which help to link the information to specific clinical scenarios.

The book is designed to be read as a whole or for the reader to dip into specific chapters. Reading all the chapters, however, will provide an excellent overview of information. The first three chapters provide prerequisite knowledge required for working with older people as a general client group, with later chapters focused on more specific theoretical and practical application. See the next section for chapter summaries.

Terminology and chapter summaries

With the aim of minimising confusion and avoiding ambiguity, the following terms will be used consistently throughout the book, although it is recognised that there are multiple synonymous or interchangeable terms.

Impairment/changes: used interchangeably to refer to typical age-related change. Although the term 'impairment' can be used with reference to a pathology or a disorder in some situations, here, it is used to refer to a normal symptom of older age but one which may cause some impairment compared with previous functioning. For example, a typical age-related hearing loss can be viewed as an impairment. The World Health Organisation (1980) refers to 'impairment' as being a loss, whether physiological or psychological, a disturbance affecting function (e.g. memory changes).

Clinician: a healthcare professional. This is generally used as a reference to any healthcare professional working with an older adult. Specific clinicians, such as a speech and language therapist or a geriatrician, will be referred to as such.

Client: a patient, a service user or anyone in receipt of services from a clinician.

Communication: refers to all aspects and methods of communication, such as speech, language, written, spoken or symbols. Certain types of communication will be specified where required.

Eating, drinking and swallowing: references all phases of the eating, drinking and swallowing process. Specific phases of the swallowing process will be referred to as such.

Older adult or older person: refers to the medical reference for an older adult; hence, any person over the age of 65.

Pathological change, disease or disorder: refers to changes related to disease or disorder rather than natural age-related changes.

The terms 'difficulties' or 'problems' may be used to explain overall communication and swallowing changes, which may be a mix of normal ageing or combined typical ageing alongside a disorder.

Summary of chapters

Following is a list of chapter summaries for chapters following this one to give a brief overview of the contents of the book.

Chapter 2: discusses the physiology of normal ageing, risk factors for severe effects of ageing, sarcopenia and frailty, preventative measures, neuroplasticity, and rehabilitation.

Chapter 3: focuses on working with older people as a client group and special considerations, including how to make the most of appointments, effects of medication, client- professional relationship, ageism and safeguarding.

Chapter 4: focuses on how ageing impacts communication. Focuses on all aspects of communication in older age, such as lifestyle changes, technology, psychological and physiological changes affecting speech and/or language.

Chapter 5: focuses on practical applications of assessing and managing communication impairment in older people. Case studies and information resources can be found at the end of the chapter.

Chapter 6: discusses the theory of how ageing affects the eating, drinking and swallowing process. Covers general changes to eating, drinking and swallowing in older age and compares the typical physiology of the swallowing phases in younger people with age-related changes.

Chapter 7: mirrors Chapter 5 but focuses on the practical applications of assessing and managing swallowing impairments in older people. Similarly, there are multiple resources and case studies that can be found at the end of the chapter.

Chapter 8: discusses decision making in older age, including advanced decision making and mental capacity. There are case studies to illustrate how the theory works in practice and practical strategies for supporting people's communication to facilitate decision making.

Chapter 9: focuses on palliative and end of life care. This chapter has more of a focus on end of life care in the last few months, weeks or days of life; how swallowing and communication is affected; and how these can be supported to ensure comfort. There is a case study and proforma of an end of life care plan at the end of the chapter.

Chapter 10: focuses on conclusion and the future. This chapter concludes the book with a look back at the main themes and a vision of how healthcare for older people with communication and swallowing impairments might look in the future.

References

Age UK (2018) *All the Lonely People: Loneliness in Later Life*. www.ageuk.org.uk accessed 8/12/2020 at 9.55.

British Geriatrics Society (2020) www.bgs.org.uk/about accessed 22/11/2020 at 12.44.

Hofman, MR et al. (2017) Elderly patients with an atypical presentation of illness in the emergency department. *The Netherlands Journal of Medicine*. 75 (6).

Kingston, A et al. (2018) MODEM project: Projections of multimorbidity in the older population in England to 2035: Estimates from the population ageing and care simulation (PACsim) model. *Age and Ageing*. 47 (3): 374–380, May 1.

Le Couteur, DG, McLachlan, AJ and de Cabo, R (2012) Aging, drugs and drug metabolism. *The Journals of Gerontology: Series A*. 67A (2): 137–139.

Lin, FR et al. (2011) Hearing loss and incident dementia. *Archives of Neurology*. 68 (2): 214–220, February.

Office for National Statistics (2020) www.ons.gov.uk/peoplepopulationandcommunity/birthsdeaths andmarriages/ageing/bulletin/estimatesoftheveryoldincludingcentenarians accessed 18/11/2020 at 14.32.

Public Health England (2018) *Health Profile for England. Chapter One: Population Change and Trends in Life Expectancy*. www.gov.uk accessed 2/5/2021 at 14.17.

Shukla, A et al. (2020) Hearing loss, loneliness and social isolation: A systematic review. Otolaryngology-head and neck surgery. *Sage Journals*. https://doi.org/10.1177/0194599820910377

Social Care Institute for Excellence (2006) Assessing the mental health needs of older people. *SCIE Guide*. 3.

Valtorta, NK et al. (2016) Loneliness and social isolation as risk factors for coronary heart disease and stroke; systematic review and meta-analysis of longitudinal observation studies, heart. *BMJ Journals*. 102 (13).

World Health Organisation (1980) *International Classification of Impairments, Disabilities, and Handicaps: A Manual of Classification Related to the Consequence of Disease*. www.who.int accessed 5/10/2021 at 12.05.

World Health Organisation (2018) *Ageing and Health*. www.who.int accessed 30/4/2021 at 14.05.

Wu, B (2020) Social isolation and loneliness among older adults in the context of COVID-19: A global challenge. *Global Health Research and Policy*. 5: 27.

PHYSIOLOGY OF AGEING, RISK FACTORS AND REHABILITATION

DOI: 10.4324/9781003058090-3

Introduction

As we journey through life, our bodies naturally start to age and decline. This decline is usually gradual and takes place over several decades but can be expedited with significant change, such as a sudden trauma, chronic illness or general lifestyle factors. Although the effects of ageing may occur in a similar pattern in all older people, the speed and the severity of ageing is heterogeneous and depends on various factors. The first sections of this chapter focus on the ways in which the brain and muscular system alter with age and ageing effects, such as reduced muscle strength and increased risk of frailty. The subsequent sections explore protective factors that can mitigate the impact of ageing, the prognostic indicators that can be used to identify people who are at risk of ageing less well and the role of neuroplasticity and rehabilitation.

The topics in this chapter are discussed in broad terms with the aim of providing a foundation of knowledge, which will then be referred to more specifically in terms of age-related changes to communication and swallowing; these are discussed in future chapters.

The ageing neuromuscular system

Atrophy of the brain occurs alongside the natural ageing process. Some sources report that this can start to happen as young as 40 years old but with increasing rate in older age (Peters, 2006). Although age-related atrophy of the brain is normal, the rate of change and the site of the atrophy can vary between individuals. These patterns of change can be a predictor of risk factors for developing conditions such as dementia. It is thought the rate of typical age-related brain atrophy is greatest in the frontal lobes with more severe cognitive changes, such as Alzheimer's disease associated with more diffuse and accelerated brain atrophy (Irwin et al., 2018).

Neuronal and chemical changes also occur with advancing age. Neurones, cells that transport information between the brain and other parts of the body via nerve impulses, reduce in size, and there is a reduction in the number of connections between the neurones (Shafto and Tyler, 2014). This can lead to slower, less targeted and reduced intensity of some nerve signals.

In terms of physical decline in normal ageing, there is a reduction in muscle mass and strength, and a reduction in bone density (Novotny et al., 2015). Waters et al. (2010) suggest that the rate of muscle loss is estimated to be at a rate of 1–2% annually after the age of 50. Whilst muscle mass and strength decreases, there is an age-related increase in body fat. This progressive loss of skeletal muscle mass is referred to as age-related *sarcopenia*, which is discussed in upcoming sections of this chapter and later in the book.

Cognitive changes are discussed in more detail in Chapter 4. Normal age-related changes to cognition include a reduction in processing speed and memory changes (Harada et al., 2013). Hearing impairment has been cited as an independent risk factor for cognitive decline (Lin et al., 2013). The diagnosable condition of mild cognitive impairment is seen as a middle ground between the normal cognitive changes of ageing, and the more severe pathological cognitive changes of dementia has increased prevalence with age (Lu et al., 2021). However, not all people with mild cognitive impairment will go on to develop dementia (Irwin et al., 2018).

Although age-related decline can be separated into physical and cognitive decline, there are clear interactions between the two with changes to brain function affecting physicality as well as cognitive function. An investigation by Auyeung et al. (2011) found association between physical frailty in cognitively normal older adults and their future cognitive decline. Loss of physical ability can lead to fewer opportunities for social interaction, which can in turn lead to cognitive decline.

Sarcopenia and frailty

'Sarcopenia' and 'frailty' are two terms that are used frequently in relation to older adults and ageing. Sarcopenia is a process involving loss of skeletal muscle fibres and reduced strength. This occurs naturally in ageing to a lesser or greater extent. Factors such as illness and poor nutrition can contribute to more severe sarcopenia, as can a period of inactivity due to a hospital admission, for example, which can lead to increased sarcopenia from deconditioning of the muscles.

The adjective 'frail' has long been used to describe older people presenting with weakness and reduced function. However, the term 'frailty' is a diagnosable medical syndrome associated with significantly more prevalence in older people. Frailty is a syndrome that affects multiple physiological systems as a result of general decline and leads to significantly increased vulnerability and reduced resilience to internal and external stressors on the body (Dodds and Sayer, 2016). As examples, an internal stressor could be an illness, such as a urinary tract infection, and an external stressor could be a bereavement.

Both sarcopenia and frailty present with similar symptoms, such as reduced muscle mass, slower ambulatory speed and reduced grip strength (Dodds and Sayer, 2016), but the effects of frailty reach deeper into the physiological systems, such as the neuromuscular, endocrine, immune, respiratory and cardiovascular systems (Clegg et al., 2013). Both sarcopenia and frailty are influenced by factors such as nutrition, mobility and overall baseline health and fitness.

Although sarcopenia is a naturally occurring side effect of the ageing process, it's progression into the realms of frailty is not considered to be an inevitable or natural part of ageing (British Geriatrics Society, 2015). Frailty can occur in people at any age but has a higher prevalence amongst older people with around a quarter of adults over 80 meeting the definition (Collard et al., 2012). It is associated with increased hospital admission, increased mortality and increased dependence for care (Vermeiren et al., 2016). Older people with frailty are, for example, more likely to develop delirium, although delirium is not as well recognised in people with frailty (Geriatric Medicine Research Collaborative, 2019).

Sarcopenia and frailty are discussed in more detail in later chapters, in particular with relation to their effect on swallowing in older age.

Cognitive and physical reserve

Despite the inevitable decline with age and the various negative consequences of this, there is reason to be positive and hopeful that the ageing process does not necessarily lead to reduced quality of life. There are a number of protective factors that contribute to a slower, less significant ageing process and which can reduce the risk of severe sarcopenia and frailty in an older person.

Accumulation of these protective factors is linked with level of reserve. In this case, 'reserve' refers to baseline levels of cognitive and physical ability. A higher level of cognitive and physical function at baseline translates into a greater reserve of these skills and greater compensation meaning that the effects of ageing might have less of an impact on overall cognitive and physical function in these cases.

A person's genetic make-up can act as a protective factor in cognitive and physical reserve in that some people are naturally predisposed to either a reduced or a more significant age-related decline (Buchman et al., 2016). There is interplay between genetic disposition and environmental factors described later that create a unique risk factor for each individual.

Studies suggest that education builds a greater level of cognitive reserve to mitigate the risk of developing Alzheimer's disease and other related dementias (Clouston et al., 2019). Other studies report that education does not affect the rate of cognitive decline in older age, although it does contribute to a higher baseline of cognitive reserve such that people in older age who were educated to a higher level will continue to function cognitively better than people in older age who received a lower level of education (Lenehan et al., 2015). Steptoe and Zaninotto (2020) link lower socio-economic status with increased pace of ageing.

Cognitively stimulating activities, such as doing puzzles, playing musical instruments and reading, can slow cognitive decline (Harada, 2013). Making use of social networks for regular interaction and emotional support is an important protective factor for maintenance of cognitive ability (Williams and Kemper, 2010), which highlights the risk of cognitive decline amongst lonely or socially isolated older people.

A good physical reserve can be built up by maintaining a level of physical fitness in the years leading up to older age with regular exercise and strength training.

Sufficient nutrient intake and weight maintenance are required for both cognitive and physical fitness. Malnutrition in older people is common and linked with poor outcomes, such as increased hospitalisation and mortality, and requires early diagnosis and intervention (Williams, 2018).

The potential for change

All the earlier topics point to an important public health message for people to maintain cognitively stimulating activities, fulfilling social networks and decent physical fitness throughout their lives to reduce the speed and severity of age-related decline (see Diagram 2.1). These factors are becoming increasingly well known, and the prospect of 'social prescribing' (clinicians linking people with community exercise or social groups) is now a welcome reality in some areas. However, many older people are still presenting at clinics with the effects of age-related decline already visible. This leads to the question of whether skills or exercise training can be used to delay further age-related decline and whether new skills can be learned and maintained.

Neuroplasticity refers to the brain's ability to reorganise and change neural pathways, and create new pathways and connections between neurones. The brain is able to navigate

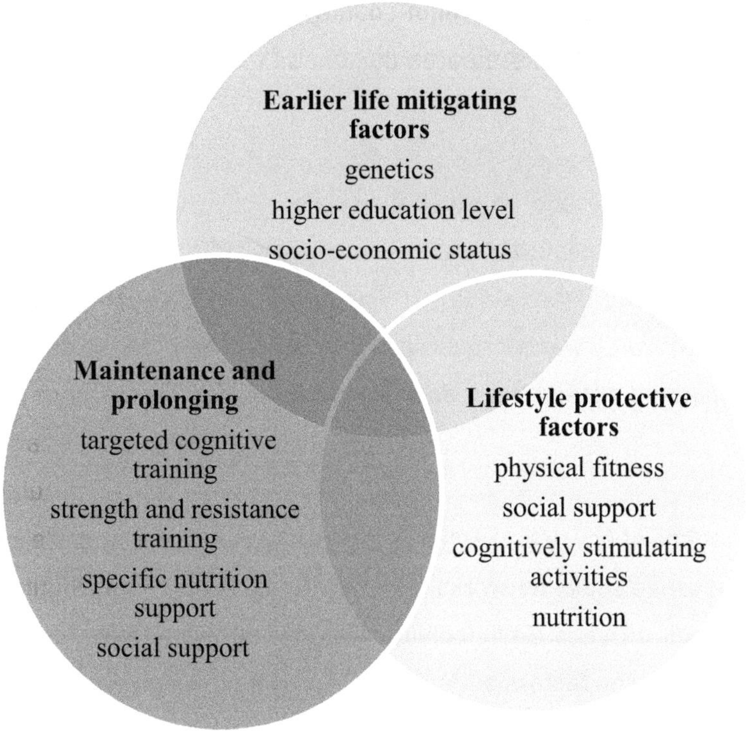

Diagram 2.1 *The interplay of factors associated with slower and less severe age-related cognitive and physical decline*

around damaged areas and recruit functioning areas to fulfil the role of the damaged areas. An example of neuroplasticity is how the brain can redirect functions to working areas of the brain during rehabilitation following brain damage caused by stroke.

It is reassuring knowledge that brain neuroplasticity can continue throughout the lifespan, allowing for the formation of new neural pathways so that older people can benefit from rehabilitation to learn new skills or to slow down further age-related decline. Cabeza et al. (2019) report that older people can compensate for decline in neural activity by recruiting from other parts of the brain. Older adults presenting with reasonable preservation of cognitive skills that are usually associated with age-related decline, such as episodic or working memory, show increased compensatory activity in the prefrontal cortex (Shafto et al., 2014).

The benefit of targeted cognitive training in older age has been found in several studies with evidence of longer-term maintenance of these skills (Williams and Kemper, 2010). There is evidence, however, that there is usually only benefit to the specific cognitive skill that was trained and that generalisation to other cognitive functions does not generally occur (Park and Bischof, 2013).

In the case of sarcopenia, strength resistance training has been found to be the most effective exercise to mitigate the effects of ageing on muscle loss and strength (Waters et al., 2010).

Nutrition plays a role in both cognitive and physical ability, and studies have cited the importance of nutrition in slowing changes with age, in particular with the role of protein consumption and vitamin D intake (Morley et al., 2010). Parsons et al. (2019) studied the diets of older men and found that frailty was more prevalent in those who followed a high-fat/low-fibre diet; those that followed a Mediterranean-style diet were less likely to develop frailty.

Continuation of or starting a regime of physical exercise, good nutritional intake, cognitively stimulating exercises and supportive social networks are, therefore, likely to contribute to slower and less pervasive changes with age. Each individual will benefit from these in their own unique way, taking into account the factors of genetics, education level and earlier life physical and cognitive fitness.

Prognostic indicators

The knowledge of the factors that can slow down or reduce the impact of age-related decline are of use in determining the prognostic indicators of older patients in terms of their risk factors for developing symptoms that have a significant impact on their quality of life.

Clinicians treating older people need to be aware of their underlying risk factors and treat these alongside the impairment itself. For example, an older person experiencing unsatisfactory levels of social interaction is at risk of developing a more significant age-related communication impairment. An older person with a poor diet and weight loss is at increased risk of sarcopenia and developing an age-related swallow impairment.

At the end of this chapter, there are proformas of a pre-assessment lifestyle questionnaire and a prognostic indicators checklist. The questionnaire can be sent out with appointment details for the client to fill in and send or email back via a secure route prior to the appointment. The clinician can then plot the risk factors onto the prognostic indicators checklist. This checklist works by ticking the factors that apply to the individual. The more ticks indicate a higher risk factor for more severe age-related decline. There is a section at the bottom of the checklist to assess the likelihood of positive response to intervention and

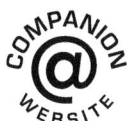

to assess what support measures might need to be put in place. Such profiles can also help with the triage of clients in a clinic to work out who is priority for intervention.

The information can be discussed with the client or family in the clinic and be used for setting functional goals. Education can be given on lifestyle factors to reduce the impact of ageing, and referrals can be made to specific clinicians if this is required. A dietitian, for example, can advise on dietary factors if the client is at risk of malnourishment. At the end of this chapter, there is also an example of an information leaflet that can be given to clients to inform them on improving lifestyle factors linked with more significant ageing.

If the client is receiving intervention for a communication disorder, for example, it makes sense that they are also working to maintain the lifestyle factors required to reduce their risk factors for age-related decline, otherwise recovery from the communication disorder can be inhibited and can be further complicated by age-related communication changes.

Chapter summary

- Normal age-related changes include atrophy of the brain, reduced neural activity and loss of muscle strength, resulting in cognitive and physical changes.
- Sarcopenia is associated with normal ageing, but there is individual variation. Frailty has some similarities with sarcopenia, but its effects are pervasive, affecting many of the physiological systems. Frailty is not associated with normal, healthy ageing but has increased prevalence with age. Frailty is associated with poor health outcomes.
- Greater cognitive and physical reserves are associated with reduced effects of ageing.
- Genetics, socio-economic status, cognitive ability, physical strength, dietary intake and social connections all play a role in how ageing affects the body.
- Neuroplasticity can continue throughout the lifespan. Older people do benefit from rehabilitation.
- Profiling of prognostic indicators can help predict which people are more at risk of serious age-related changes.

Resources

- Pre-assessment profile (Table 2.1)
- Prognostic indicators checklist (Table 2.2)
- Lifestyle changes to reduce the impact of ageing on quality of life (leaflet for clients or carers)

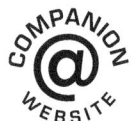

Pre-assessment profile

This can be sent to the patient by post along with the appointment details or given as an electronic copy following a booking via telephone call. This can be made in large print.

Table 2.1 Pre-assessment profile

Pre-assessment lifestyle questionnaire
Name: DOB: Occupation or previous occupation, if applicable? *If you are retired, please give the date of your retirement.* Hearing ability: Visual ability: Current medication (please also detail any side effects):
Social and emotional
• Have there been any recent lifestyle changes (e.g. moving house or bereavement)? • How do you feel about social activities? • Has your enjoyment of social activities improved, gotten worse or stayed the same? Please indicate why. • What kind of social activities are you involved with? • How often are you able to be involved in social activities? • Is there anything that prevents you from joining in with social activities (e.g. communication difficulties, tiredness, low confidence and transport)? • Do you have regular interactions, either face to face or over video/phone call, with other people? • Do you feel your social/family networks offer you emotional support when required? • How often do you feel lonely or low?
Activities
• Do you do have any hobbies (e.g. music, books or crossword)? • Is there anything that prevents you being able to enjoy your hobbies (e.g. poor eyesight)? • How much physical exercise are you able to do? • What sort of physical exercises do you do? • Is there anything that prevents you from being able to take part in physical exercise? • Do you feel physically weaker than you used to? If so, how does this affect your lifestyle?
Nutrition
• Are you able to visit the shop for food and drink? • Are you able to cook your own meals? • If not, who provides these for you? • Do you have any dietary restrictions or do you avoid certain foods? • Do you feel you are able to eat a balanced diet? • Do you enjoy eating out? • Have you experienced any weight loss recently?
Hopes and goals
• What is most important to you in your life at the moment in terms of your quality of life? • What do you feel would improve your lifestyle at the moment? • What do you hope to get out of your upcoming appointment?

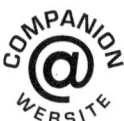

Prognostic indicators checklist

Table 2.2   Prognostic indicators checklist (adapted from Martin (2021) *Working with Voice Disorders: Theory and Practice, 3rd edition. Appendix VII*)

Prognostic indicator	Tick if present
Medical comorbidities	
Medication side effects affecting quality of life	
Hearing impairment	
Visual impairment	
Social and emotional support	
Mood changes?	
Limited or no social and/or family networks	
Limited or no hobbies and activities	
Physical factors	
Weakness/frailty	
Reduced or no physical exercise	
Nutrition	
Poor diet	
Avoidance of certain foods	
Inability to prepare meals	
Factors influencing response to intervention	Yes/No
Does the current impairment significantly affect lifestyle?	
Will the patient receive positive support: From family/significant others?	
Is the patient motivated?	
Are patient/family expectations realistic?	
Has the patient had treatment for a similar impairment before?	
Was it successful?	

Lifestyle changes to reduce the impact of ageing on quality of life

Several changes occur in our bodies because of the natural ageing process. As part of this process, you may have noticed changes, such as difficulty finding words at times, slower processing of information or slightly weaker muscles.

The speed and severity of age-related decline is an interplay between genetics and lifestyle factors. Detailed subsequently are some guidance and ideas for improving lifestyle factors related to age-related change. Applying these suggestions can help to slow down and reduce the impact of ageing on your body and mind.

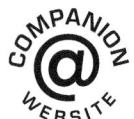

Physical exercise

Taking part in regular exercise can help to reduce age-related weakness both physically and cognitively. There may be exercise groups in your area that are designed for older adults.

It is thought that strength resistance exercises are especially beneficial to people in older age.

Nutrition

Eating a balanced diet helps to optimise how the body works and, therefore, minimise certain nutritional deficiencies that can lead to a more noticeable age-related physical and cognitive decline.

If you are overweight, have unintentional weight loss, are struggling to prepare meals or feel as though you are not able to get a balanced diet, you may need to make some changes. Speak to your doctor for further advice. A referral to a dietitian may be required.

Cognitive

Engaging regularly in cognitively challenging and social activities can help towards slowing age-related decline.

Activities such as reading, playing a musical instrument, playing jigsaws or crossword puzzles can help.

Participating in social activities and engaging in regular conversations can also help with maintaining cognitive and communication skills. There are usually local social activities or befriending schemes that can be accessed.

> If you notice symptoms are getting worse, for example, increased frequency of word finding difficulty and increased muscle weakness, or if you develop symptoms, such as memory loss or swallowing difficulties, please consult your doctor for further investigation.

References

Auyeung, TW, Lee JSW and Woo, J (2011) Physical frailty predicts future cognitive decline- a four year prospective study in 2737 cognitively normal older adults. The Journal of Nutrition, Health and Aging. 15 690-694.

British Geriatrics Society and Royal College of General Practitioners in Association with Age UK (2015) Fit for Frailty Part 2: developing, commissioning and managing services for people living with frailty in community settings. A report.

Cabeza, R et al. (2019) Cognitive neuroscience of healthy aging: Maintenance, reserve and compensation. *Nature Reviews Neuroscience.* 19 (11): 701-702, November.

Clegg, A et al. (2013) Frailty in elderly people. *The Lancet.* 381 (9698): 752-762.

Clouston, SAP et al. (2019) Education and cognitive decline: An integrative analysis of global longitudinal studies of cognitive ageing. *The Journals of Gerontology: Series B.* 75 (7): e151-e160.

Collard, RM et al. (2012) Prevalence of frailty in community dwelling older persons: A systematic review. *Journal of American Geriatrics Society.* 60 (8): 1487-1492.

Dodds, R and Sayer, AA (2016) Sarcopenia and frailty: new challenges for clinical practice. Clinical Medicine (London) Oct: 16 (5).

Geriatric Medicine Research Collaborative (2019) Delirium is prevalent in older hospital inpatients and associated with adverse outcomes: Results of prospective multi-centre study on world delirium awareness day. *BMC Medicine.* 17: 229.

Harada, CN, Natelson Love , MC and Triebel, K (2013) Normal Cognitive Aging. Clinical Geriatric Medicine. Nov 29 (4) 737-752.

Irwin, K et al. (2018) Healthy aging and dementia: Two roads diverging in midlife? Review article. *Frontiers in Aging Neuroscience.* 19.

Lenehan, ME et al. (2015) Relationship between education and age-related cognitive decline: A review of the recent research. *Psychogeriatrics.* 15 (2): 154-162.

Lin, FR et al (2013) Hearing loss and cognitive decline in older adults. JAMA Internal Medicine 173(4): 293-299.

Lu, Y et al. (2021) Prevalence of mild cognitive impairment in community dwelling Chinese populations aged over 55 years: A meta-analysis and systematic review. *BMC Geriatrics.* 21: 10.

Martin, S (2021) *Working with Voice Disorders: Theory and Practice.* 3rd Edition. Routledge Publishers.

Morley, J et al (2010) Nutritional recommendations for the management of sarcopenia. Journal of the American Medical Directors Association Jul 11 (6): 391-396.

Novotny, SA, Warren, GL and Hamrick, MW (2015) Aging and the Muscle-Bone relationship. Physiology (Bethesda) Jan; 30 (1): 8-16.

Park, D and Bischof, G (2013) The aging mind: neuroplasticity in response to cognitive training. Dialogues in Clinical Neuroscience 15(1): 109-119.

Parsons, TJ et al. (2019) Physical frailty in older men: Prospective associations with diet quality and patterns. *Age and Ageing.* 48 (3): 355-360.

Peters, R (2006) Ageing and the brain. *Postgraduate Medical Journal, BMJ.* 82 (964): 84-88, February.

Shafto, M and Tyler, L (2014) Language and the aging brain; the network dynamics of cognitive decline and preservation. *Science.* 346 (6209): 583-587.

Steptoe, A and Zaninotto, P (2020) Lower socioeconomic status and the acceleration of aging: An outcome-wide analysis. *Proceedings of the National Academy of Sciences of the United States of America.* 117 (26): 14911-14917.

Vermeiren, S et al. On behalf of the Gerontopole Brussels Study Group (2016) Frailty and the predictions of negative health outcomes. A meta-analysis. *Journal of Post Acute and Long Term Care Medicine, Online Review Article.* 17 (12): 1163.E1-1163.E17.

Waters, DL et al. (2010) Advantages of dietary, exercise related, and therapeutic interventions to prevent and treat sarcopenia in adult patients: An update. *Clinical Interventions in Aging.* 7 (5): 259-270.

Williams, S (2018) Improving nutrition to support healthy ageing: What are the opportunities for intervention? *The Proceedings of the Nutrition Society.* 77 (3): 257-264, August.

WORKING WITH AN OLDER CLIENT GROUP

DOI: 10.4324/9781003058090-4

Introduction

This chapter moves on to focus on the practical aspects of working with older people as a client group. It contains information, advice and strategies to enable the clinician to be flexible and responsive to the needs of their older clients in order for both older clients and clinicians to get the best out of their clinical encounters.

Individual considerations

The ability to tailor a clinical service to each client's individual needs is desirable but often needs to be balanced with the constraints of the service provision and organisational demands. There are, however, several ways in which the clinician can use their knowledge to work flexibly in these contexts in order optimise the experience of each client and, ultimately, the outcome of their work together.

Some of these considerations are discussed subsequently.

Hearing and visual impairments

Older people more commonly experience hearing and/or visual impairments than those in young or middle age (see next chapter for more detail). It is important for the clinician to be aware of the impact of these and to make necessary adjustments to accommodate. For example, choose a quiet room with little background noise, avoid telephone conversations where hearing is an issue and provide written information in larger print.

Fatigue

Older people commonly report feelings of fatigue (Moreh et al., 2010). The processing of information, learning new skills and putting these into practice will take more effort, especially when there are compounding factors, such as hearing and/or visual impairments.

Journeying to the hospital or clinic and locating the room venue might mean that the client arrives at the appointment already with some level of fatigue. Clients living on their own or those who do not speak frequently with other people may find interaction tiring initially. Fatigue levels need to be observed and discussed with the client. Consideration must be given to the environment and timing of the appointment and the client's usual circumstances. Assessment scores may not be accurate if the client is fatigued above their usual level. Assessments may be repeated, but it needs to be acknowledged that there may be a priming effect from the first assessment that could inflate scores.

Where possible, there should be flexibility with the timings of appointments, pacing of activities in the session and a short break in the middle of the session if beneficial. An older client may benefit from arriving ten minutes earlier for a session and resting in the waiting room before entering the appointment.

Side effects of medication

As mentioned in the introductory chapter, the body responds to and metabolises medication differently as it ages. Many older people regularly take several medications (known as polypharmacy), which increases the risk of side effects or adverse effects (Cantlay et al., 2016).

Common medications in the elderly include anticholinergic medication, prescribed for a range of conditions, such as bladder problems and chronic obstructive pulmonary disease (Grossi et al., 2020). The side effects of this class of medication include drowsiness, dry mouth, dry eyes and reduced cognitive function (Kouladjian O'Donnell et al., 2016).

Other common side effects of medication in the elderly include fatigue and confusion.

Significant side effects will have an impact on both communication and swallowing (see later chapters for more detail) and quality of life. Symptoms such as confusion and fatigue will affect the ability to participate in assessment and therapy. Of course, the benefits of the medication need to be weighed up against the impact of extra symptoms caused by the medication on general lifestyle and function.

It is always worthwhile to ask the client about any symptoms that could be related to their medication and ask them to visit their doctor to discuss this further if there are concerns.

Learning styles

Learning styles broadly fall into categories. There are differing opinions of how many learning categories exist, but four that are often cited are described here:

- Visual: learning best from information presented in images, charts or graphs.
- Auditory: learning best from hearing information.

- Reading and writing: reading text or writing information down.
- Kinaesthetic: learning best through interactive or sensory learning environment.

(Fleming and Mills, 1992)

Willingham et al. (2015) argue that a learning style is a personal preference of modality through which to process information rather than a heightened ability to receive information in a particular form. Some people challenge the notion of a learning style and view it as a reflection on an individual's belief of best learning style rather than how they actually process information (Krätzig et al., 2006). Nonetheless, it is useful for the clinician to be aware of each client's preference of learning modality so that they can adapt the way that they present information to optimise the client's retention and use of the information given.

Older people are likely to be aware of their own learning preference and will either be able to communicate this or identify their style from a choice of examples. Their belief about their own learning preference is likely to have become embedded over many years, which can make it more challenging for them to receive information in less preferred ways.

Normal age-related cognitive changes need to be taken into account when considering how older people take on information. These cognitive changes will be discussed in greater detail in the next chapter, but it has been noted that older people have reduced processing speed, can be less flexible in their thinking and tend to respond better to concrete examples rather than abstract concepts (Harada et al., 2013).

Written material to take away from the session can reduce the burden on the client of having to remember what has been said and advised. Kessels (2003) suggests that written information is more easily remembered and cites several reasons that older people might have difficulty recalling verbally presented clinical information, including reduced short-term memory, anxiety and distress, and discordance of information with client's previously held beliefs about a particular health issue or disease.

Motivations and expectations

Gauging the motivation of a client to attend clinic for assessment or to seek therapy is useful as it provides a good benchmark from which to plan realistic goals. Knowledge of the referral pathway offers insight into this and can be asked in the initial session. Was it the client who initiated the referral or a concerned family member? Other questions to explore initially are whether the client would be motivated to do work at home between sessions and what it would mean for them if their communication and/or swallowing ability improved.

The prognostic indicators checklist in Chapter 2 is a useful tool from which to gain some background information.

The motivation or expectations of an older client might be influenced by their own beliefs and assumptions about ageing. In some older people, there might be the underlying belief that it is too late to access treatment or that they will not be able to learn new skills. There might be some fear around a medical diagnosis and what they believe this might mean for them. Being aware of beliefs that present as a barrier to the client's progress helps them to be discussed in a sensitive and empathetic manner with reassurance from the clinician.

Expectations of the intervention can be openly discussed so that the clinician and client can realistically plan and agree individualised goals. Is the client expecting an official medical diagnosis from the first appointment? What are they expecting in terms of recovery for their communication and/or swallowing difficulties? What type of intervention are they expecting in terms of timings and frequency?

What one person hopes to achieve from their treatment and what is important to that individual might be very different from another individual with the same impairment. For instance, one person with symptoms of swallowing difficulty might have a goal that links to their desire to eat out socially whilst another person with the same symptoms might be wanting general education and advice. For this reason, treatment and goal planning need to be person centred and outcome measures to be broad and flexible enough that they capture the qualitative benefit to the individual. Goal planning and outcome measures with respect to communication and swallowing will be discussed in more detail in later chapters.

Table 3.1 is a summary of the factors discussed that are beneficial to have in mind when working with older people and strategies to support these in clinical encounters.

Table 3.1 Summary of individual considerations

Individual considerations	Strategies to support
Hearing and/or visual impairment	Ask the client what helps Choose a quiet room Avoid telephone calls if hearing is a problem Provide large print written material for visual impairment
Fatigue	Talk to the client about their experience of fatigue Adjust timing of appointment if possible Pace activities Break down assessments and activities into shorter sections if possible Consider that fatigue may reduce the accuracy of assessment scores

Individual considerations	Strategies to support
Medication side effects	Talk to the client about any symptoms that might be due to medication side effects (e.g. drowsiness, confusion, dry mouth and dry eyes)
	Ask the client to talk to their doctor/GP if the side effects are significantly impacting on access to assessment and therapy or the client's quality of life
Learning styles	May be more embedded in older people
	Learn how your client prefers information to be presented
	Allow for age-related effects, such as slower processing speed and better ability to process concrete rather than abstract concepts
	Provide written material to help the client remember information, strategies or exercises
Motivation and expectation	Use the prognostic indicators checklist from Chapter 2
	Discuss expectations with the client
	Set realistic and individualised goals

Clinician-older-client relationship

Building an effective rapport

Giving time and effort to building rapport with clients reaps benefits in the positivity of client experience, satisfaction and health outcomes (Williams et al., 2007).

The clinician is often called to build this rapport quickly in the context of time and resource pressures, and it is a skill that requires experience and reflection but also leads to a great deal of satisfaction on the behalf of the clinician as well as the client.

Skills that support effective rapport building include active listening, focused concentration on what the client is saying and use of non-verbal language that reflects engagement, such as leaning forward, nodding or paraphrasing. Listening and interaction should take place with empathy and without judgement. The clinician needs to understand and be sensitive towards clients' cultural and spiritual needs.

Most clinicians are taught these valuable skills in their training, and the use of role play and video feedback are useful tools in cultivating rapport-building skills.

Language style or elderspeak

It has been noted that some people adopt a particular style of spoken interaction when addressing older people. This has been termed 'elderspeak' by researchers.

Elderspeak has many characteristics, including a slower rate of speech, higher pitch, increased volume and reduced grammatical and word complexity (Williams et al., 2009). The researchers also found increased use of collective pronouns – the use of 'we' in place of 'you' – for example, 'Shall we take this medication now?'.

Elderspeak is often adopted due to perceived incompetence of conversational ability in older adults. It tends to be used with good intentions to facilitate the communication of older adults in conversation. Kemper and Harden (1999) analysed whether there were any aspects of elderspeak that were beneficial to the communication of older adults and found that reducing grammatical complexity and complexity of meaning did facilitate conversation but that characteristics, such as slowing speaking rate and reducing sentence length, were not helpful.

But evidence has found that older people react negatively to being addressed with elderspeak, with it being perceived as patronising and giving a feeling of incompetence (Williams et al., 2005).

The paradox in which people believe they are helping by using elderspeak and older people feeling patronised can impact negatively on relationships. Williams et al. (2009) found a link between the use of elderspeak by staff members and residents' resistance to receiving care in care homes for people with dementia.

It has been found that making people aware of their use of elderspeak and of older people's perception of elderspeak is beneficial. A randomised control trial in which staff in dementia care homes were made aware of their use of elderspeak through a training programme reduced the frequency of its use (Williams et al., 2017).

As with developing skills for relationship building, the use of role play, video feedback and feedback from clients and colleagues will help clinicians become more aware of their use of elderspeak with the aim of reducing it.

Dynamics within the relationship

It is important to be aware of factors that can affect the dynamic of the relationship between clinician and older patient. Clients will have had varying experience of medical settings and will vary in their perception of health professionals. Eliassen (2016) writes that medical professionals are assumed to have more power than their clients in terms of medical expertise and knowledge of health systems. Some older clients, either culturally or generationally, will view health professionals with reverence and feel unable to question their authority. Other clients may have had an unpleasant experience in the past, leading to a fear of healthcare settings.

A clinician needs to have sensitivity to the potential power dynamics, listen to client's stories and perceptions, and try to make sure that power dynamics do not interfere with treatment or decision making. The use of technical medical language, which can alienate clients and interfere with decision making, needs to be avoided, as well as the use of any acronyms or younger vocabulary that an older person may not understand.

Ageism

Clinicians have a duty to examine their own beliefs and judgements about older age and the provision of healthcare for older people, and to challenge any ageism that presents in their own actions or those of people or organisations. Older people should not be denied or given any lower provision of healthcare due to their age alone. Such actions are illegal in the UK (BMJ, 2012).

Holistic management

It has been observed that older people are less likely to discuss psychosocial issues within medical appointments (Williams et al., 2007). This may be due either to thoughts that it is not an appropriate topic for medical settings or a discomfort in initiating these conversation topics.

However, when these issues are raised, it leads to a more effective professional relationship, with the clinician treating the client more holistically and being able to choose the most effective treatment for that client and their particular circumstances, as well as signposting to other services that might be of help.

A client is unlikely to be able to engage fully with treatment if they are concerned about their living or financial circumstances. Therefore, the onus is on the clinician to enquire sensitively about emotional and psychosocial circumstances during their interactions. The depth of these conversations will vary depending on the setting and reason for appointment.

Decision making

When the clinician seeks to make decisions collaboratively with the client, there is more likelihood of the client adhering to the treatment plan (Williams et al., 2007). The older client is likely to feel more listened to and invested in their treatment if they have been able to contribute to decision making and goal planning. This involves a meeting of and flexibility within the clinician's expectations and clinical evidence base with the client's expectations and life circumstances. A solution-focused approach (Burns, 2016) is an effective way of harnessing the older client's wisdom and choices about what is important in terms of quality of life.

Presence of a third party during the appointment

Older people are often accompanied to the clinic by another person, either a family member or friend. This can alter the dynamic of the professional relationship and the experience of the older person in different ways. It has been found that older people do not raise as many topics and are less responsive in terms of asking questions or clarifying when there is a third party present in the appointment (Williams et al., 2007). Older clients might defer to the accompanying person to ask and answer questions rather than do so themselves or the other person might feel the need to talk for them. Clinicians can navigate this by asking and clarifying issues with the client directly rather than the other person.

It can, however, be helpful to have a third party in the clinic room, especially when it comes to recalling what has been said at the appointment or to asking questions. Attending clinic with another person can also be a source of support and comfort for an older person.

If the client does not have English as their first language, then the third person in the room could act as a translator. This might be a professional translator or a family member. In the case of this being a family member, it needs to be remembered that direct translation of what the clinician or the client has said might not be achieved due to the family member relaying their own understanding, summarising or paraphrasing. A professional translator is more reliable with accuracy of translation, but the client may still prefer to have a family member present.

Ending of the professional relationship

The relationship with the clinician may be the most prominent relationship in the older person's life and act as a source of social and emotional support, as well as addressing medical matters. For older people with communication difficulties, they may feel that their clinician is the only person who can understand them and facilitate their communication.

Awareness of this will help the clinician to plan for the end of the treatment and think about who or what might support the client in future. Engaging family or friends in therapy with the client's consent can model how to support the client's communication and help them to learn and practise communication strategies. It is useful to explore options outside the clinic settings, such as volunteer organisations, befriending schemes and social groups, that the client can be signposted to or supported in joining. If the clinician suspects that the client may require more emotional support, the client can be supported to seek a referral for more targeted professional help.

As discussed, the nature of the relationship between the clinician and the older person is such that advance planning for the time when the assessment or treatment plan ends is critical. This event needs to be discussed with the client in advance or in plenty of time so that preparations can be made and expectations managed. It is good to talk about feelings surrounding this event and to provide support dealing with this change, particularly if the client has been receiving long-term intervention.

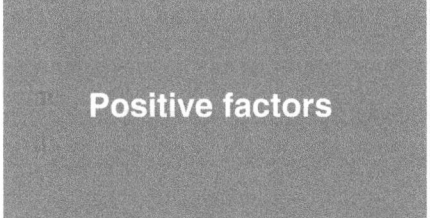

Positive factors

- Active listening
- Empathy and non-judgement
- Discussion of psycho-social topics
- Shared decision making
- Sensitivity towards the impact of third-party presence
- Planned, careful ending of the professional relationship

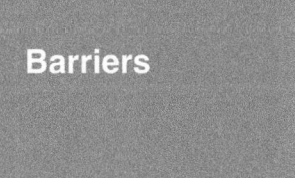

Barriers

- Elderspeak
- Ageism
- Unequal power dynamic
- Clinician-led decisions
- Avoidance of psycho-social topics
- Reduced awareness ofthe potential impact of third-party presence
- Abrupt, unplanned ending

Diagram 3.1 *Positive factors and barriers involved in creating a strong and effective older person–clinician relationship*

Safeguarding and older people

All clinicians need to be alert to any signs that are suspicious of their clients being subject to abuse from another person or signs that abuse might be occurring within the client's close circle.

Unfortunately, this is no less the case when working with older people. The World Health Organisation (2020) estimate that one in six older people globally are subject to some form of abuse. In fact, this is thought to be a significant underestimate, as they believe that only around a quarter of cases of abuse against older people are reported. Abuse can relate to a single event or a neglect, or ongoing events that cause any harm or distress to a person or compromise human rights (WHO, 2020). The World Health Organisation (2020) predicts an increase in elder abuse in future years, arising from a growth in the elderly population and reduced resources domestically and institutionally to meet their needs.

Older people can be more vulnerable to abuse. Changes such as physical frailty and cognitive decline can lead to increased dependency on other people, which can in turn lead to situations in which patterns of abuse can arise. Older people with communication difficulties are also likely to be more vulnerable to ill treatment or to be taken advantage of as they are less able to report what is happening.

Abuse can take several forms, including physical, financial, sexual, emotional and neglect. The most common form that older people are subjected to is thought to be emotional or physical neglect. Examples of this include not changing an older person's clothes when they are dirty, not giving sufficient choices or sufficient independence to make decisions, or not attending to a person when they are clearly in distress. Cases of abuse are thought to be more prevalent in institutional rather than community settings (WHO, 2021). This is especially the case where staff training is poor and where standards for the older person and their care workers are low.

Abuse can also occur within the home. Changes to relationships in which one person becomes more dependent on another can precipitate this. Domestic abuse is also prevalent within the older population with Age UK reporting that 23% of victims of domestic homicide are over the age of 60 (Age UK, 2019).

A clinician has a duty to report any suspected abuse and to be aware of the structures in place within the organisation on how to report and/or to seek advice from senior colleagues. All conversations should be taken seriously with sensitivity to the older person's situation but with clinicians making it clear that they have a duty to report this information if it is disclosed. Clinicians need to be aware that an older person might not recognise that they are being subject to abuse or be fearful of the consequences of reporting such issues.

People with communication difficulties may be more likely to divulge possible abuse to clinicians who are supporting them with their communication difficulty, such as a speech and language therapist. The SLT can facilitate their communication to help them express their views more clearly or more coherently with the SLT being mindful of not asking leading or presumptuous questions. An SLT can act as a communication facilitator or provide a summary of how best to communicate with a person with communication difficulties who is reporting possible abuse.

Chapter summary

- Clinicians benefit from offering flexibility to their older clients to meet their individual needs in order for them to get the best out of the clinical intervention. Older people may have different needs to their younger counterparts.

- Clinicians cultivating an effective professional relationship with older clients will benefit both the client and clinician. Barriers to creating an effective rapport include elderspeak and negative beliefs about age.

- All clinicians have a duty to be vigilant about signs of abuse and to report any suspicions or disclosures in line with the safeguarding policy of their organisation. Older people with communication difficulties may require the support of an SLT to communicate their concerns.

References

Age UK (n.d.) www.ageuk.org.uk/latest-press/articles/2019/october/at-least-200000-older-people-experienced-domestic-abuse-last-year-but-the-experiences-of-over-75s-are-being-entirely-overlooked/ accessed 24/10/2019 at 15.42.

British Medical Journal (2012) Age discrimination in UK healthcare will become unlawful in October. *BMJ*. 344-4134.

Burns, K (2016) *Focus on Solutions: A Health Professional's Guide*. 2nd Edition. Solution Books.

Cantley, A, Glyn, T and Barton, N (2016) Polypharmacy in the elderly. *InnovAIT: Education and Inspiration for General Practice, InnoVAIT*. 9 (2): 69-77.

Eliassen, AH (2016) Power relations and health care communication in older adulthood: Educating recipients and providers. *The Gerontologist*. 56 (6): 990-996.

Fleming, ND and Mills, C (1992) Not another inventory rather a catalyst for reflection. *To Improve the Academy*. 11: 137-155.

Grossi, CM et al. (2020) Increasing prevalence of anticholinergic medication use in older people in England over 20 years: Cognitive function and ageing study I and II. *BMC Geriatrics*. 20: Article number 267.

Kemper, S and Harden, T (1999) Experimentally disentangling what's beneficial about elderspeak with what's not. *Psychology and Aging*. 14 (4): 656-670.

Kessels, RPC (2003) Patients' memory for medical information. *Journal for the Royal Society of Medicine*. 96: 219-222.

Kouladjian O'Donnell, K et al. (2016) Anticholinergic burden: Considerations for older adults. *Journal of Pharmacy Practice and Research*. 47 (1): 67-77.

Krätzig, GP and Arbuthnott, KD (2006) Perceptual learning style and learning proficiency: A test of the hypothesis. *Journal of Educational Psychology*. 98 (1): 238-246.

Moreh, E, Jacobs, JM and Stressman, J (2010) Fatigue, function and mortality in older adults. *The Journals of Gerontology: Series A.* 65A (8): 887-895.

Williams, K, Kemper, S and Hummert ML (2005) Enhancing communication with older adults: Overcoming elderspeak. *Journal of Psychosocial Nursing and Mental Health Services.* 43 (5): 12-16.

Williams, K et al. (2009) Elderspeak communication: Impact on dementia care. *American Journal of Alzheimer's Disease and Other Dementias.* 24 (1): 11-20.

Williams, K et al. (2017) A communication intervention to reduce resistiveness in dementia care: A cluster randomised control trial. *The Gerontologist.* 57 (4): 707-718.

Williams, SL, Haskard, KB and DiMatteo RB (2007) The therapeutic effect of the physician- older patient relationship: Effective communication with vulnerable older patients. *Clinical Interventions in Aging.* 2 (3): 453-467.

Willingham, DT, Hughes, EM and Dobolyi, DG (2015) The scientific status of learning style theories. *Society for the Teaching of Psychology.* 42 (3): 266-271.

World Health Organisation (WHO) (n.d.) www.who.int/news-room/fact-sheets/detail/elder-abuse accessed 24/10/2021 at 15.28.

COMMUNICATION IN THE CONTEXT OF OLDER AGE

DOI: 10.4324/9781003058090-5

Introduction

The ability to communicate effectively is a basic and essential human need. The reasons why we communicate are wide ranging and incorporate building and maintaining relationships, making requests and expressing emotions. The methods of communication are various and include verbal, non-verbal, written, signs and symbols.

Communication needs and methods of communication change throughout a person's lifespan. Older adults may be required to adapt their communication style in later life, for example, to accommodate altering social networks, changing lifestyles and new technologies. In parallel, they could also be navigating some of the gradual changes to communication abilities that naturally occur with ageing or a sudden significant change due to disease.

Clinicians working with older people may notice symptoms, such as voice changes and language impairments. This is especially true of professionals, such as speech and language therapists, who are trained to be highly attuned to a person's communication ability. People in older age might be unaware of the gradual changes to their communication, but a more vigilant older person or family member might notice these changes and become concerned of an underlying pathology.

It will be obvious in some cases that communication impairments are the result of a disease process, for example, following neuroimaging that confirms a stroke. However, it remains important that clinicians are aware of what symptoms of communication change represent typical ageing processes and what symptoms could be more concerning. This knowledge will equip clinicians to be able to provide reassurance to a concerned client or family member, or to have the confidence to discern when a referral for specialist assessment might be indicated. Having a gauge of what would be considered normal in ageing will also aid the clinician and client in setting realistic goals for rehabilitation.

This chapter addresses the factors that can affect communication ability later in life. It is divided into sections exploring various aspects of communication change, beginning with environmental and psychological factors, natural age-related changes and communication change associated with a pathological process.

The information in this chapter is designed to give a comprehensive overview of each of the topics and a summary of the evidence base. The aim is for a clinician to be able to use this resource confidently in clinical or learning settings, but it may also serve to ignite interest to study some of the topics in even more detail.

Environmental and psychological changes

Lifestyle changes

As people journey into older age, the communication environment of an individual can change dramatically.

Changes in important relationships brought about by loss of friendships, divorce or death of a partner can result in the breakdown of familiar, comfortable use of language and interactional patterns. These differences to people's communication life can result in fewer opportunities for fulfilling, effective communication networks as well as contribute to the decline of functional communication skills. The Office of National Statistics in the UK report a statistically significant increase in the number of older people living alone between 2008 and 2018, with 3.9 million of older people living alone in 2018 (ONS, 2019).

Another significant moment of change often occurring in older age is the event of retirement. Although the official age for retirement is increasing, so also is the age that people are living to, which means that an older person can expect to spend many years in retirement. Whether retirement is welcome or unwelcome, sudden or gradual, it is inevitable that there will be a fundamental change to a person's communication network. There will be fewer opportunities for casual conversation with colleagues, reduced need for the language and vocabulary of business, and potentially, reduced need to communicate via technology.

Changes in role, identity or relationship status can result in loss of confidence and self-esteem, leading to reduced effort and ability to create new networks. A proportion of older people have a full-time caring role, which reduces their opportunity for interaction with a variety of people. The presence of a communication disorder, such as aphasia or dysarthria, is likely to impact significantly on an older person's communication networks and their ability to create new ones.

Evidence shows that reduced participation in social, interactive and cognitive activities in later life can expedite cognitive decline (James et al., 2011), with associated effects on language ability.

It is, however, important to note that older age can also bring new opportunities and the possibility of new communication networks, and many older people continue to have effective and fulfilling communication networks. People can join new social groups, take up new hobbies, learn new skills and embark on travel. New relationships and friendships can form, and grandchildren may arrive, unleashing new opportunities for interaction.

Technology

Technology has become a vital means of communication, and people who are currently in older age will have witnessed a huge shift in technological advances across their lifespan. Technology is changing frequently and can be used for communication in multiple ways.

Technology can facilitate life in older age, with the option of online shopping or money management, as well as enabling communication with friends or relatives who do not live nearby. It has been of significant benefit to those people who have communication or sensory disorders in the form of predictive text, voice-activated software and other assistive devices.

There has been a general judgement that older people may be more reluctant to adopt new technology or have difficulty learning how to use it, and unfortunately, this can impact on an older person's self-perception or confidence in using new technology.

There is some evidence that older people are less frequent users of the internet, but use in older age is becoming more frequent. In the UK, the percentage of people between 65 and 74 years who had recently used the internet increased from 52% in 2011 to 83% in 2019 (ONS, 2019). A report from OFCOM indicates that 81% of adults over the age of 75 years use a mobile phone (OFCOM, 2019).

The recent COVID-19 pandemic has prompted many older people into learning how to use technology to connect with family members or friends when the option to see them face to face was removed. Telehealth and telemedicine have been discussed in health services for many years as a way to increase efficiency and to reach people who live more remotely but has become routinely used in the face of the pandemic when face-to-face appointments have presented a risk of catching the virus.

There is a spectrum of attitudes amongst older adults in relation to the uptake of new technology or telehealth, which have shown both positive and negative attributes (Cimperman et al., 2013). Positive attitudes include a willingness to learn and satisfaction with the ease of accessing information. The more negative attitudes and perceived barriers include comparison with younger age groups, concerns that instructions might be too complex, lack of confidence and fears about security.

If there is a judgement of older people not being as able to take on new technology, then the evidence disputes this. A large review and analysis of data of the use of telehealth with older people who have chronic heart failure showed that it was actually a very small percentage (3%) of older people who were unable to competently learn or use health technology (Clark, 2018).

Even if technological interaction is embraced and used well, it is important to remember that these cannot fully replace the value of real-life, face-to-face human interactions.

Psychological factors

Later life can bring along traumatic events and major lifestyle adjustments, such as bereavement, serious medical diagnosis, living with chronic illness or moving into residential care. These changes can have an impact on an older person's psychological health or contribute to an exacerbation of pre-existing mental ill health.

A study by McCombe et al. (2018) reviewed records from a large database and found that just over a quarter of people aged 80–84 years had a mental health disorder, with the most common of these being depression, anxiety, and alcohol and substance misuse.

The World Health Organisation (2017) states that a quarter of deaths from self-harm are from people aged 60 and above, citing risk factors, including bereavement, decline in abilities or loss of socio-economic status.

Mental ill health can have a direct impact on communication ability. There is evidence of change in speech rate (Buyukdura et al., 2011) and dry mouth (Gholhami et al., 2017). Evidence links alcohol misuse with cerebellar damage, which can lead to ataxic dysarthria (Fitzpatrick et al., 2008).

The link between antidepressants and extrapyramidal symptoms has been researched and is known that these symptoms can occur as side effects across different classes of antidepressants and at different doses (Madhusoodanan, 2010). Extrapyramidal symptoms are multiple, but many of these symptoms, such as ataxia, dyskinesia, hypertonia and Parkinsonism, will affect intelligibility of speech.

Self-perception is an additional psychological factor to consider. It is unfortunate that alongside positive messages about people being healthier in older age, able to work longer and live for longer, people are also exposed to negative societal stereotypes about ageing.

Internalisation of these stereotypes and the person's own view of ageing from their family or personal experience can contribute to negative self-perception in ageing. Interaction styles, such as elderspeak (see Chapter 3), can result in negative self-perception and feeling infantilised.

Studies have evidenced that having negative self-perception in older age is linked to negative health outcomes, including increased rates of hospitalisation (Sun et al., 2017). Levy et al. (2004) found that positive self-perception correlates to increased engagement in preventative activities, such as social groups, exercise and attendance at routine health screenings.

Physiological changes to communication in normal ageing

This second section of the chapter moves on to studying physiological processes in the ageing body, which contribute towards natural communication changes in healthy older adults (see Table 4.1). Of course, there will be some overlap and interplay with the factors discussed in the first section of the chapter, for instance, with psychological factors affecting both mind and body. Some of the processes here will affect both communication and swallowing, but these will be discussed in detail in reference to swallowing impairments in Chapter 6.

The extent to which the physiological changes impact on an ageing individual is likely to reflect the severity of their overall ageing process.

Oral health

Receding gums, damage to tooth enamel and dry mouth are common oral symptoms in older adults (Medline Plus, 2020).

As well as dry mouth being a known side effect of some medications, it has been found that quantity and quality of saliva reduces in older age (Xu et al., 2019)

The need for denture wearing also increases with age. Experiencing dry mouth or discomfort from teeth or dentures is likely to have some impact on the comfort and confidence of communicating, particularly with unfamiliar people. The effect of loose or ill-fitting dentures on articulation precision could lead to reduced intelligibility of speech.

Presbyopia

Presbyopia is a term used to describe the changes in eyesight that occur naturally with ageing. The lens of the eye begins to stiffen in the ageing process. This leads to trouble focusing on small print and on nearby small objects. Communication can be affected in terms of difficulty accessing written material. Reading glasses or contact lenses help correct this problem.

It is estimated that around 1.8 billion people globally have presbyopia (Fricke et al., 2018). It can be further complicated by other age-related visual conditions, such as macular degeneration, glaucoma and cataracts.

Presbyacusis

Presbyacusis refers to the normal loss of hearing that is associated with ageing. This is a sensorineural hearing loss and occurs along a spectrum of severity but can lead to complete functional bilateral hearing loss. There are multiple factors involved in the severity of the hearing loss, including genetic predisposition and amount of exposure to very loud noise.

Hearing loss can have a marked impact on the ability to communicate effectively and comfortably. Words and meanings can be missed, and it takes more effort to listen and participate in conversations, especially in the presence of background noise. Hearing loss has been linked with loneliness, isolation and reduced psychological wellbeing (Ciorba et al., 2012). As previously mentioned, it has been found that older people with hearing loss are at increased risk of developing dementia.

Hearing loss can be rehabilitated somewhat by the use of hearing aids, and in some cases, cochlear implants are considered.

Breath support for voice and speech

Lung capacity starts to decline approximately after the age of 35 (American Lung Association, 2021), although the severity and speed of this depends on general health, genetics, exercise habits and exposure of the lungs to toxins.

During the normal ageing process, there is a reduction of respiratory muscle strength and a stiffening of the ribcage through calcification alongside reduced chest wall compliance (Sharma and Goodwin, 2006). The diaphragm is also thought to be affected by age-related sarcopenia (Greising et al., 2018).

Age-related kyphosis is related to compression or cracking of spinal bones as a result of weakness. The changing shape of the spine because of kyphosis can alter the shape of the thoracic space and lead to increased effort when breathing (Katzman et al., 2011).

The consequences of ageing effects on the respiratory system can lead to increased respiratory challenge when speaking and a subsequent reduction in breath support for effective voice production and speaking.

Articulation

Opinions differ as to how the oro-motor structure and function change in healthy ageing. There are claims that the oro-motor system in healthy older adults does not show functional decline and that oral movements, such as those of the soft palate, remain functional for speech production (Hooper and Cralidis, 2009).

An investigation by Bilodeau et al. (2015) found that speech and oro-motor control decline in accuracy with increasing age. They hypothesised this was due to factors such as reduced muscle strength, reduced efficiency of neural mechanisms or related brain changes.

The musculature related to articulation is likely to be at risk of sarcopenia with increasing age. It could be hypothesised that older people who are isolated and do not have much opportunity for spoken interaction could be at increased risk of reduced muscle strength or reduced precision of articulation.

As mentioned previously in the chapter, dentition or dentures can affect articulation, and dysarthria can be a side effect of some psychiatric medicines.

That said, unless there is an issue with dentition or dentures or a side effect of medication, a discernible dysarthria is an unusual symptom in a healthy older adult and would serve as a flag for further investigation.

Voice

Physiological effects of ageing can impact on voice quality. Martin (2021) engages in a detailed discussion of the effects of ageing on the vocal tract and voice quality in *Working with Voice Disorders (3rd edition)*. This is summarised subsequently:

- Weakening of the laryngeal muscles, calcification, and ossification of cartilages of the larynx.

- Degeneration of cells in the mucous membranes leading to a drying effect.
- Breakdown and reduced thickness of the elastic fibres in the vocal ligament.
- Weakening of neural innervation to the vocal cords causing reduced vocal cord approximation.
- Lower fundamental frequency of the male voice with increasing age
- Mixed views on whether there is significant change to the female fundamental frequency post menopause.

The impact of ageing on the respiratory system, such as reduced ribcage movement (see earlier in the chapter), can result in reduced breath support for voice production.

As a result of these changes, the ageing voice may sound more breathy, weak or dry. Older males will tend to present with a somewhat higher voice than younger males.

Vocabulary and word retrieval

Older adults frequently report word finding difficulty or the tip-of-the-tongue phenomenon as a symptom that appears to increase with age (Burke and Shafto, 2004). This can lead to frustration, reduced confidence or concern about the possibility of an underlying reason, such as an early symptom of dementia.

The bank of vocabulary that a person has stored appears to remain stable or gradually increases throughout life, along with experience and exposure to different words (Harada et al., 2013). It is thought that access to the meaning of words (semantic representations) does not generally decline, or at least does not until very old age, in healthy older people (James and Burke, 2000).

Although semantic representations of words seem to remain robust in older age, it is thought that ageing reduces the strength of the connection between the semantic representations (representations of meanings) of words and phonological representations (sound representation) of words. Speech errors that occur in older age are more likely to be sound errors, such as 'pin' instead of 'pig', rather than errors of meaning, such as 'pencil' instead of 'pen'. Burke and Shafto (2004) describe this in terms of the transmission deficit model in which there is insufficient activation of the phonological representation of the word due to weak connections from the semantic system. Part of the word might be retrieved, such as the first sound, if there is partial activation. There is a frustrating tip-of-the-tongue phenomenon in which the person knows the word they want to say and can often think of the first sound, but the rest of the word does not come easily. Burke and Shafto (2004) note that these errors are more likely to be present in older age and more likely to occur on words that the person uses less frequently, as the brain is less practised at retrieving these words.

It has been observed that healthy older people make more errors on confrontational naming tasks, such as picture naming, than they do in general conversation. Zec et al. (2005) found that confrontational naming ability starts to decline approximately after the age of 70. Confrontational naming tasks are, however, more challenging than connected, spontaneous speech, with the extra demands of assessment and reduced semantic and phonological context.

Although presumably, older people are referring to connected, spontaneous speech when they report word retrieval difficulty, there have been studies that suggest word retrieval errors are not common in connected speech in healthy older people. A review by Kavé and Goral (2017) compared studies relating to word retrieval errors in connected speech and tested them against four hypotheses – reduced verbal output, reduced lexical diversity, increased word retrieval behaviours and an association between tests of single-word production and word retrieval errors in context. They found insufficient evidence to support any of these hypotheses within the healthy ageing population.

Even though this evidence appears to suggest fewer word retrieval errors in connected speech, word retrieval difficulty remains a frequently reported symptom in healthy older age, and reassurance or strategies can be given to support these symptoms (see Chapter 5). It is also necessary for the person to monitor word retrieval difficulties and to seek further investigation if they become more frequent or occur alongside other symptoms, such as memory loss.

Verbal fluency

Verbal fluency is a measure of word retrieval from a specific semantic or phonological category within a specified time frame. A semantic category might be naming types of animals, and a phonological category could be naming words beginning with the letter *s*.

Verbal fluency draws on both executive control and language skill. However, there has been conflicting opinion and multiple studies about what this task is actually testing and what it can divulge about specifics of a person's cognitive or language ability, which are difficult to tease apart (McDowd et al., 2011). However, tests of verbal fluency are routinely included in tests that are used to evaluate the cognitive skills of older people, and therefore, it has been included here.

It is generally agreed that there is a decline in verbal fluency with healthy ageing and a more noticeable decline in semantic fluency (Gordon et al., 2017). Slower lexical retrieval speed is thought to be a factor in this decline (Gordon et al., 2017; McDowd et al., 2011). Higher verbal fluency scores have been linked with educational level in healthy older people (Charchat-Fichman et al., 2009) and, therefore, should be considered when interpreting scores.

Grammar

Syntactic structure of sentences is not thought to be affected by ageing. Research indicates that healthy older people produce less grammatically complex sentences than their younger counterparts (Kemper et al., 2003).

Comprehension and auditory processing

It can be difficult to separate and assess comprehension of spoken language alongside competing factors, such as reduced hearing ability and processing speed.

Processing of language becomes slower in healthy older people (Tun et al., 2012). Comprehension of language may be more difficult out of context, and there appears to be a priming effect in that older people can be more suggestive to given examples or leading questions, which in turn can influence their responses (Bryan and Maxim, 2006).

It is generally accepted that comprehension of spoken language in older age is functional unless task demands or conversational complexity are particularly challenging and/or there is an uncorrected hearing impairment (Worrall and Hickson, 2003).

Cognitive skills

Although cognitive skills have been discussed here in the context of language, it is noted that there is a natural decline in other cognitive skills during the process of ageing.

Harada et al. (2013) give a comprehensive account in their review of studies into the effects of ageing on cognition. They report a gradual decline in fluid intelligence, such as executive functioning, psychomotor ability, processing speed and learning, but a stability of crystallised intelligence, such as vocabulary knowledge and general knowledge.

As far as memory is concerned, Harada et al. (2013) report poorer performance on memory tasks in healthy older adults compared to younger adults. Rönnlund et al. (2005) report that episodic memory (memory of previous experiences) declines throughout the lifespan, whereas semantic memory (e.g. practical knowledge and information) starts to decline only in later life.

Conversational skills

Conversational skills in older age can be troublesome to qualify, as conversation skills in themselves vary between people, and much depends on an individual's baseline conversational style.

Older people use more words in conversation, and there is an increase of talk drifting away from the topic of conversation (off-topic verbosity) associated with ageing (Arbunkle et al., 2004). In Arbunkle and colleagues' study, it was found that high level of off-topic verbosity was associated with decline in daily activities and a subsequent association with loneliness. They also acknowledge that off-topic verbosity can be a signal of motivation of desire to interact with others. Smith et al. (2019) also found a link between off-topic verbosity and loneliness. However, people will respond to loneliness differently, and some people may not speak as much.

Off-topic verbosity in older age has been linked with age-related cognitive decline with reduced inhibitory processes, meaning reduced ability to filter out irrelevant information and slower verbal set shifting (e.g. moving from one topic to another) (Barnett and Coldiron, 2021).

Older adults use increased ambiguous pronoun references in conversation, which can lead to the listener having trouble keeping track of whom the speaker is referring to. Hendriks et al. (2014) studied the use of ambiguous pronouns in older adults and claimed this is due to reduced cognitive capability to keep track of the referents.

Of course, conversation efficacy can be affected by other factors discussed previously in the chapter, such as poor hearing, conversational complexity and word retrieval difficulty, and psychological factors, including reduced confidence and poor self-perception.

Reading

Reading ability to can be affected by visual impairment in older age. Changes to the lens in the eye described earlier in the chapter make it increasingly difficult to read smaller print. This can be corrected by using glasses or making the print larger.

Levels of fatigue or reduced concentration or attention are also likely to have an impact on reading ability, particularly with more complex or unfamiliar reading material.

There is some evidence that older people can become more sensitive to spatial frequency in text, which can affect reading ability (Paterson et al., 2013).

Writing

Writing in older age can be more challenging if there are visual impairments or with conditions, such as arthritis, affecting the physical action of writing. Burke and Shafto (2004) found evidence to support their hypothesis that the tip-of-the-tongue phenomenon reported in the speech of older people can also occur with spelling, as there are weaker connections from the semantic representation to the orthographic (written) representation of words. Therefore, word retrieval difficulty can occur with written words as well as spoken in older age.

Summary

Table 4.1 Summary of what are considered typical age-related changes to communication

Visual changes	Difficulty accessing written material, especially small print.
Hearing changes	Difficulty participating in conversation, missing words and meanings.
Respiratory system	Reduced breath support for voice and speech production.
Articulation	No discernible effects due to ageing, but poor dentition or loose dentures can affect intelligibility of speech.
Voice	Voice quality can change. The voice can become weaker and breathier sounding. Reduced breath support can affect voice production.
Word retrieval	Can be more evident in picture-naming tasks than in connected speech, although is a frequently reported symptom. Phonological errors are more common than semantic errors.
Verbal fluency	Declines in older age. Declines are more evident in semantic category naming.
Comprehension	Compounded by poor hearing, slower processing speed, task demands and conversational complexity. Priming effects. Comprehension of spoken language generally functional.
Auditory processing	Slower in older age.
Grammar	Generally remains intact. Some evidence of reduced production of grammatically complex sentences.
Cognitive skills	Decline of fluid intelligence (e.g. executive functioning, processing speed and psychomotor ability). Stable crystallised intelligence, such as vocabulary and general knowledge. Semantic memory declines in later life whilst episodic memory declines throughout life.

(Continued)

Table 4.1 (Continued)

Visual changes	Difficulty accessing written material, especially small print.
Conversation	Increased use of ambiguous pronouns. Increased frequency of off-topic verbosity.
Reading	Affected by visual changes. Increased sensitivity to spatial frequencies may affect reading in older age. Other factors affecting reading ability include reduced concentration and fatigue.
Writing	Affected by visual changes and other physical changes, such as arthritis. Word retrieval difficulties can be present in writing as well as speech.

Pathological changes to communication in ageing

There are several diseases that are more prevalent in older age for which deterioration in communication ability is a significant symptom and that clinicians will routinely come across in their work. Listed in Table 4.2 are some of the most common of these diseases, although not an exhaustive list. There are various resources widely available for each of these diseases, and clinicians are invited to access these to read further about ones of particular interest. For the purposes of this book, clinicians need to be aware that alongside the disease-related communication impairment, there will be an overlay of age-related communication impairment for older clients.

In the next chapter, there is a table on differential diagnosis of communication symptoms that can appear in older age and what these symptoms might indicate for underlying pathology. There is a spectrum of severity of communication symptoms in normal older age, making it difficult to quantify what exactly is normal. As will be addressed in the next chapter, some of these normal age-related changes might also be masking early symptoms of a more serious disorder, such as a dementia.

Table 4.2 List of diseases in which communication difficulties commonly present as a symptom

Diseases with communication impairment as a likely symptom
Benign voice pathology
Head and neck cancer
Stroke
Dementia
Delirium
Mild cognitive impairment
Progressive neurological diseases (e.g. motor neurone disease, Parkinson's disease and related diseases, and cortico-basal degeneration)
Head injury
Brain tumour
Mental illness

Chapter summary

- Communication in older age can be influenced by lifestyle changes, technology and psychological factors.

- There are physiological changes occurring with age, alongside the previously mentioned factors, which impact on several areas of communication, such as processing speed, voice production, word retrieval and grammatical complexity.

- The extent of age-related communication change will vary between individuals, depending on the overall severity of age-related change in that individual.

- There is a higher prevalence of diseases in older age for which decline in communication ability is a significant symptom.

References

American Lung Association (n.d.) www.lung.org accessed 19/5/2021 at 20.47.

Arbuckle, TY et al. (2004) Off topic verbosity: Everyday competence, and subjective wellbeing. *Gerontology*. 50: 291-297.

Barnett, M and Coldiron, AM (2021) Off topic verbosity: Relationships between verbal abilities and speech characteristics among young and older adults. *Applied Neurology: Adult*. https://doi.org/10.1080/23279095.2021.1878461

Bilodeau-Mecure, M et al. (2015) Movement frequency in normal ageing: Speech, oro-facial and finger movements. *Age*. 37: 78.

Bryan, K and Maxim, J (Eds) (2006) *Communication Disability in the Dementias*. Whurr Publishers Limited.

Burke, D and Shafto, M (2004) Aging and language production. *Current Directions in Psychological Science*. 13 (1): 21-24.

Buyukdura, JS, McClintock, SM and Croarkin, PE (2011) Psychomotor retardation in depression: Biological underpinnings, measurement and treatment. *Progress in Neuro-Psychopharmacology and Biological Psychiatry*. 35 (2): 395-409, March 30.

Charchat Fichman, H et al. (2009) Age and educational level effects on performance of normal elderly on category verbal fluency tasks. *Dementia and Neuropsychologia*. 3 (1): 49-54.

Cimperman, M et al. (2013) Older adult's perceptions of home telehealth services. *Telemedicine Journal and E-Health*. 19 (10): 786-790, October.

Ciorba, A et al. (2012) The impact of hearing loss on the quality of life of older adults. *Clinical Interventions in Aging*. 7: 159-163.

Clark, RA (2018) Telehealth in the elderly with chronic heart failure: What is the evidence? *Studies in Health Technology and Informatics*. 246: 18-23.

Fitzpatrick, LE, Jackson, M and Crowe, SF (2008) The relationship between alcoholic cerebellar degeneration and cognitive and emotional functioning. *Neuroscience and Biobehavioural Reviews*. 32 (3): 466-485.

Fricke, T et al. (2018). Global prevalence of presbyopia and vision impairment from uncorrected presbyopia: Systematic review, meta-analysis and modelling. *Ophthalmology*. 125 (10): 1492-1499.

Gholami, N et al. (2017) Effect of stress, anxiety and depression on unstimulated salivary flow rate and xerostomia. *Journal of Dental Research, Dental Clinics, Dental Prospects*. 11 (4): 247-252, Autumn.

Gordon, J, Young, M and Garcia, C (2017) Why do older adults have difficulty with semantic fluency? *Aging, Neuropsychology and Cognition*. 25 (6).

Greising, SM et al. (2018) Diaphragm plasticity in aging and disease: Therapies for muscle weakness go from strength to strength. *Journal of Applied Physiology*. 125 (2): 243-253.

Harada, C, Natelson Love, M and Triebel, K (2013) Normal cognitive aging. *Clinical Geriatric Medicine*. 4: 737-752, November 29.

Hendriks, P, Koster, C and Hoeks JCJ (2014) Referential choice across the lifespan: why children and adults produce ambiguous pronouns. Language, Cognition and Neuroscience 29:4 391-407.

Hooper, CR and Cralidis, A (2009) Normal changes in the speech of older adults: You have still got what it takes, it just takes a little longer! *Perspectives on Gerontology*. 14 (2): 47-56.

James, B et al. (2011) Late-life social activity and cognitive decline in old age. *Journal of International Neuropsychological Society*. 6: 998-1005, November 17.

James, L and Burke, D (2000) Phonological priming effects on word retrieval and tip of the tongue experiences in young and older adults. *Journal of Experimental Psychology: Learning, Memory and Cognition*. 26 (6): 1378-1391.

Kavé G and Goral, M (2017) Do age related word retrieval difficulties appear (or disappear) in connected speech? Neuropsychology, Development and Cognition. Section B, Aging, Neuropsychology and Cognition Sept 24(5): 508-527.

Katzman, WB et al. (2011) Age-related hyperkyphosis: Its causes, consequences and management. *The Journal of Orthopaedic and Sports Physical Therapy*. 40 (6): 352-360.

Kemper, S et al. (2003) Age differences in sentence production. *Journal of Gerontology. Series B, Psychological Sciences and Social Sciences*. 58 (5): 260-268.

Levy, BR and Myers, LM (2004) Preventative health behaviours influenced by self-perceptions of ageing. *Preventive Medicine*. 39: 625-629.

Madhusoodanan, S et al (2010) Extrapyradimal symptoms associated with antidepressants- a review of the literature and analysis of spontaneous reports. Annals of Clinical Psychiatry Aug 22 (3): 148-56.

Martin, S (2021) *Working with Voice Disorders: Theory and Practice*. 3rd Edition. Routledge.

McCombe, G et al. (2018) Identified mental disorders in older adults in primary care; a cross-sectional database study. *European Journal of General Practice*. 24 (1): 84-91.

McDowd, J et al. (2011) Understanding verbal fluency in healthy older aging, Alzheimer's disease and Parkinson's disease. *Neuropsychology*. 25 (2): 210-225.

OFCOM (2019) *Adults: Media Use and Attitudes Report*. https://ofcom.org.uk/_data/assets/pdf-file/0021/149124/adults-media-use-and-attitudes-report.pdf accessed 25/4/2020.

Office for National Statistics: Internet Users UK (2019) www.ons.gov.uk/businessindustryand trade/itandinternetindustry/bulletins/internetusers/2019 accessed 29/3/2020 at 15.30.

Office for National Statistics (n.d.) www.ons.gov.uk/peoplepopulationandcommunity/birthsdeathsandmarriages/families/bulletins/familiesandhouseholds/2019 accessed 9/5/2020 at 15.53.

Paterson, KB, McGowan, VA and Jordan, TR (2013) Effects of adult aging on reading filtered text: Evidence from eye movements. *PeerJ- Life and Environment*. 1: e63.

Rönnlund, M et al. (2005) Stability, growth and decline in adult life span development of declarative memory: Cross sectional and longitudinal data from a population-based study. *Psychology and Aging*. 20: 3-18.

Sharma, G and Goodwin, J (2006) Effect of aging on respiratory system physiology and immunology. *Clinical Interventions in Aging*. 1 (3): 253-260.

Smith, LN et al. (2019) Ramble on: Loneliness and off topic verbosity in older adults. *Innovation in Aging*. 3 (Suppl 1): S531.

Sun, J, Kim, E and Smith, J (2017) Positive self-perceptions of ageing and lower rate of overnight hospitalisation in the US population over 50. *Psychosomatic Medicine*. 79 (1): 81-90.

Tun, PA et al. (2012) The effects of ageing on auditory processing and cognition. *American Journal of Audiology*. 21 (2): 344-350.

Medline Plus National Library of Medicine (2021) Aging changes in teeth and gums https://medlineplus.gov accessed 24/4/22 at 15.06.

World Health Organisation (n.d.) www.who.int/news-room/fact-sheets/detail/mental-health-of-older-adults accessed 28/3/2017.

Worrall, L and Hickson, L (2003) *Communication Disability in Aging: From Prevention to Intervention*. Delmar Learning.

Xu, F, Laguna, L and Sarkar, A (2019) Age related changes in the quality and quantity of saliva: Where do we stand in our understanding? *Journal of Texture Studies*. 50 (1): 27-35.

Zec, RF et al. (2005) A longitudinal study of confrontation naming in the 'normal' elderly. *Journal of the International Neuropsychological Society*. 11: 716-726.

CLINICAL ASSESSMENT AND MANAGEMENT OF COMMUNICATION IN OLDER ADULTS

DOI: 10.4324/9781003058090-6

Introduction

Following on from the previous chapter, which focused on theory and evidence relating to communication changes later in life, this chapter will discuss the practical application of this knowledge in clinical settings.

This chapter will assist the clinician in building a skill set for working with older people with communication impairments. It follows through a typical clinical journey, from case history taking, assessment and interpretation, goal setting, intervention, outcomes and follow-up. There are case scenarios to demonstrate these skills in practice and resources for clinicians at the end of the chapter.

In keeping with the premise of the book, the information is broad and generic but easily applicable and adaptable for various aetiologies, and includes specific ideas and considerations that are relevant and important for older clients.

Clinical journey

Pre-appointment information

Although a communication screen may be carried out by another professional, it is the speech and language therapist who will carry out the full assessment and intervention for a communication impairment. It is often worthwhile to gather some information about the client's communication concerns prior to the initial appointment. There can be little detail on the referral letter, which can make it difficult to triage the urgency of the appointment.

The prognostic indicators checklist at the end of Chapter 2 is useful to give an overall picture of the client's individual risk factors for experiencing more significant age-related effects. At the end of this chapter, there is a communication symptoms checklist that can be filled in by the client or a family member. This brief screen of symptoms can help the clinician to determine the urgency of appointment based on the symptoms and whether they point to age-related change or to a possible serious underlying cause. They can also help the client to be more aware of their communication and the specifics of the difficulties being experienced.

These resources can be sent out in an initial contact letter to the client and requested that they are securely emailed back before an initial appointment is made. Alternatively, these sheets could be given out to the main referrers to the Speech and Language Therapy team in order to gain more detail about the symptoms prompting the referral and to aid with triage.

Case history

Obtaining a detailed case history is essential clinical practice for all new clients to any clinical setting. Information from the case history helps the clinician to start to form hypotheses about the nature and severity of the presenting issue, and informs decision making as to the next steps. If the right questions are asked, it also helps the clinician to form a holistic view of the impairment and the effect of it on the client's wellbeing.

This practice of gathering information can also provide a valuable language sample for the clinician who can informally begin to assess the client's speech and language at the same time. If the client has moderate to severe communication problems, the clinician can use supportive resources, such as alphabet charts or pictures. A family member can also help provide some of the information.

An example proforma of a case history for older people presenting with communication impairment can be found at the end of this chapter in the 'Resources' section. Some sections of the case history proforma and the rationale behind the questions are discussed subsequently.

Baseline communication style

What is or used to be the client's usual communication style? This is pertinent information, especially if the clinician is assessing whether the communication impairment is age-related or pathological. Communication style varies significantly from person to person, and it is the level of deviation from the client's normal communication style that generates cause for concern. For example, a person who was usually social and enjoyed talking who is now not being as socially active would be cause for concern.

Sleep habits or energy levels

It is useful to have this information about an older client. Sleep habits often change as a person gets older, and daily activities change. Insomnia and early morning waking are common. Having an awareness of your client's energy levels throughout the day can inform the time that you make their next appointment to maximise engagement and learning potential. Sudden changes in sleeping habits or energy levels, or experiences of very low energy levels without an adequate explanation would prompt a referral to the doctor for further investigation. These can be linked with mood changes or possible underlying disorders.

Smoking status or alcohol intake

Both smoking and alcohol intake increase the risk of developing cancer and other diseases. The risk of developing cancer and other disease is already heightened due to the age of the client. Information on smoking frequency and alcohol consumption is essential to know to be able to signpost to support services, if required, or to be aware that this person may be at increased risk of illness, such as head and neck cancer.

Recent lifestyle changes

Later life can bring lifestyle changes that can impact significantly on an older person. Examples include a move to a new house to be closer to family, a move to a care home or a bereavement. These changes will take time to process and acclimatise to, and could also expedite age-related decline if the right support is not in place. Awareness of these changes help the clinician assess the client and the impairment in the context of their current lifestyle circumstances.

Accuracy of information

Looking from the client perspective, it can be daunting to be asked questions by someone you have just met for the first time, even if it is a health professional. The client may not feel comfortable divulging information to begin with but might become more open as the sessions progress. It is not unusual for older people be fearful of the potential consequences of mentioning symptoms, such as memory problems due to anxiety around the possibility of cognitive impairment or dementia.

Assessment

The next task that follows from case history taking tends to involve some sort of assessment. This can take many forms depending on the nature of the impairment and the type of clinic. Consideration needs to be given to the context in which the assessment is delivered in order to give clients the best chance of showing an accurate reflection of their ability. Variables are discussed in the interpretation section. Various forms of assessment are detailed subsequently:

Screening assessment

In order to gain insight into the client's full communication ability, it is prudent to carry out a language screening assessment with each client. A client may have been referred with a particular concern, such as a word finding difficulty or a more obvious symptom, but a comprehensive screening assessment might also pick up some more subtle comprehension difficulties. A screen can be particularly useful when working with older people to gain a baseline measure of their overall communication ability. It can start to signal to the clinician whether the client is presenting with normal age-related decline or not. For instance, it would raise some concern if the client was not able to follow simple spoken instructions out of context (allowing for hearing difficulty), as this is not considered within normal limits of age-related decline.

Screening assessments typically tend to be quite short and easy to administer. They can be easily replicated so the clinician can check any changes in language ability over time and can also help the clinician to decide which areas require further assessment. If the service allows, it may be less taxing for the client to have a case history and screening assessment at the first appointment and a more targeted assessment at a subsequent appointment.

There are various language screening tests that are widely used in hospital and clinical settings. Some settings will have developed their own for use in their settings, and the choice is also often down to clinician preference based on usability and experience. So long as the screening tool covers all aspects of language, including expressive and receptive language, both verbal and written, then it will provide a comprehensive measure of a person's language ability. The same screening tool should be used for the same client for repeat assessment to check progress or to compare current ability to baseline ability.

Formal versus informal assessment

Clinicians tend to use a mixture of formal and informal assessment to assess a particular language area. It is imperative to note that there is little normative data available for older people given the heterogeneity of age-related decline, and therefore, standardised scoring might not have been validated for older people.

Following is a summary of the advantages and disadvantages of formal and informal assessments when working with older people.

Formal assessment

Advantages

☑ Detailed instructions about how to use
☑ Reliable baseline measure of impairment
☑ Easy to replicate under similar circumstances
☑ Structured scoring

Disadvantages

☒ Standardisation/normative scores might not be validated for normal age-related decline
☒ Assessment can be longer and more complicated, contributing to fatigue
☒ Formality of assessment might be stressful for an older person, and this could affect scoring

Informal assessment

Advantages

☑ Gives a more natural language sample
☑ Gives more flexibility with administering
☑ Can be less stressful for an older person
☑ Is often shorter than a more formal assessment

Disadvantages

☒ Not as easy to replicate
☒ Less structured and may not measure all levels of impairment
☒ Less standardised scoring

Interpretation

Interpretation of assessment scores needs to be cautious and to take into account a number of factors. As mentioned previously, a standardised assessment that relates scores to normative data might not accommodate normal age-related decline. If there is an age range within the standardised scores, then this will give a more accurate picture.

The context in which the assessment was carried out could impact on assessment scoring. Did the client appear tired during the assessment? Did the client appear anxious? In some cases, the assessment will take place whilst the client is an inpatient in the hospital. If clients are dehydrated or acutely unwell with an infection, their ability to focus their attention on assessment could well be affected, and their cognitive and communication abilities might be temporarily worse than usual, making age-related symptoms more prominent. This is not necessarily a reflection of their abilities when they are fit and well.

Language samples in a clinical setting irrespective of whether the assessment is formal or informal may not be representative of the client's language in real-life situations.

Sometimes, observation of the client informally conversing with a family member can offer valuable insight.

Other factors that might skew results are the presence of other symptoms. For example, a person with short-term memory problems might have difficulty with some of the assessment, but that does not necessarily reflect language impairment. Conversely, many of the formal cognitive assessments that are routinely used in healthcare settings have sections on picture naming and verbal fluency. A person with a pre-existing language disorder, such as aphasia, might have low scores on these, but that does not necessarily reflect a cognitive impairment.

A skilled clinician will gather information from the case history, informal conversation with the client and assessment scores, and use this evidence to form hypotheses and plan intervention. Although it is understood that some assessments will be a one-off meeting and the clinician will have to form a hypothesis on the basis of this, most hypotheses are evolving, and the clinician will gather more information as the relationship develops with the client.

The clinician must have in mind whether this language impairment is typical for old age or whether it could be something more concerning. This is no easy task, as there is little normative data and age-related decline occurs on a spectrum of severity. Gathering as much information as possible can aid the clinician in their decision making. As therapists become more used to working with older people, they can develop a sense of what is typical. Student clinicians benefit from placement experience of communicating with older adults in a general setting, such as a care home.

Referring back to the case history and prognostic indicators status can give clinicians a clue as to whether this is a typical language decline of older age. For example, for someone who does not have so much opportunity for conversation, one would expect a more marked age-related decline in language, but for someone who frequently engages in conversation, one would expect there to be less age-related decline, as communication skills are being practised regularly. Similarly, if there were additional symptoms alongside language decline (e.g. short-term memory problems), this would warrant further investigation.

Sometimes a client will need to be reviewed over a period of time to check the rate and pattern of language decline.

A clinician may feel that it is appropriate to explore differential diagnosis if there are other symptoms or if there is uncertainty over whether the communication symptoms are age-related or not.

Table 5.1 sets out some examples of such scenarios and from whom to seek further investigation. Where and how to seek further investigation will vary depending on local services. In the UK, the general practitioner (GP) is often the person who will initiate referrals following requests from the clinician.

Table 5.1 Some examples of scenarios and from whom to seek further investigation

Symptom	Possible underlying causes	Further investigation / from whom to seek referral
Persistent, deteriorating unusual voice quality (e.g. hoarseness and breathiness) **Red flags: smoking status and alcohol intake**	• Voice disorder • Head and neck cancer • Progressive neurological disease	Ear, nose and throat specialists in the first instance
Apparent sudden onset of impaired speech and/or language **Red flags: dysarthria, aphasia or dysphagia**	• Stroke • Transient ischaemic attack (TIA) • Brain haemorrhage	Emergency services as soon as possible after onset GP for further investigation and referral for neuroimaging if there was no intervention after the event
Progressive symptoms that are affecting daily activities **Red flags: associated dysarthria, dysphagia or limb weakness**	• Progressive neurological disorders	Neurology
Reduced social interaction, reduced motivation and fearful for future **Red flags: recent lifestyle change and history of mental ill health**	• Mood changes • Mental health disorder	Psychological services
Cognitive symptoms alongside communication impairment, such as short-term memory problems, affecting daily activities **Red flags: acute infection and progressive cognitive symptoms**	• Mild cognitive impairment • Dementia • Delirium	GP for treatment if infection present Old age psychiatry Memory clinic Neurology

Goal setting

Goal setting needs to be a joint process between client and clinician, with clients leading on their own goals and clinicians helping to formulate these in terms of achievability, time frame and activities. Setting goals helps to provide a focus for sessions, manage expectations and provide a measure to track progress. Person-centred goals are important and are more likely to result in the patient's adherence to treatment. They also help to individualise treatment. Clients with severe communication difficulties might have difficulty communicating their goals and might need support in the form of pictures or symbols. If they are not able to use pictures, clinicians and family can observe and make inferences on what is important.

Although there are different ways of writing and setting goals, the SMART (specific, measurable, achievable, realistic and timely) acronym remains popular and easy to use.

Goals will differ depending on the type of impairment, the individual person and the setting. For example, the wishes of a person with a communication impairment and who is in the hospital might be different from a person receiving six outpatient sessions for communication therapy.

Here are some examples of patient goals.

> Client with delirium in hospital:
>> Goal: For the client to learn how to request a drink using an object, picture or spoken word by the end of the speech and language therapy session.
> Client with long-term severe aphasia in hospital with an infection:
>> Goal: For all ward staff working with the client to be able to use his communication book to support his communication by the end of the week
> Client with mild age-related word finding difficulties seen in outpatient clinic:
>> Goal: For the client to learn and use strategies to facilitate word finding by the end of two speech and language therapy sessions.

Intervention

Intervention very much depends on what the client goals are as well as the outcome of assessment, aetiology and prognosis. Intervention will vary widely according to the evidence base for that particular impairment and will rely on creativity and flexibility on the behalf of the clinician to balance clinical evidence base with the client's own goals and quality of life (see Diagram 5.1).

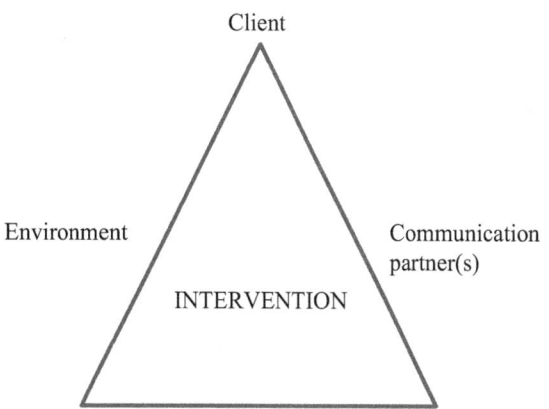

Diagram 5.1 *Considerations when deciding on appropriate communication intervention*

Intervention will be talked about in general terms here, with advice for working with older people that can be generalised across different aetiologies and health settings. The term 'intervention' is used here but could equally be called treatment or therapy.

At the end of the chapter, there are various resources that clinicians can use as part of their toolkit when working with older patients.

Intervention needs to be patient centred and individualised, as mentioned earlier. The nature of the intervention will vary. It might be impairment based, in which the client is given exercises with the aim of directly improving the impairment, such as with rehabilitation exercises following a stroke.

It may be about teaching the client to use strategies to support their communication. It could target a particular area of communication, such as improving communication on telephone calls for an older person whose family lives away or writing a birthday card to a friend.

The environment

Work with the client and/or their family member or carer to consider aspects of their environment that could change to facilitate communication. These changes could be very simple, such as reducing background noise or changing the position of the chairs in the room. This can be especially important in new settings for the client, such as a hospital setting or a care home. You may have the opportunity to work with staff in a care home to set up a designated quiet room with soft furnishings to promote effective communication for important conversations. Whilst there will be several aspects of these environments that will not be able to change, there will be some small changes that can be made to the benefit of facilitating communication.

The communication partner

Effective communication relies on successful interaction between people. This includes the ability of the people in the conversation to be able to adapt their language style to meet the language ability of the other person in the conversation and to be able to navigate, repair and move on from communication breakdowns.

The client can change communication through impairment-based work and conversational strategies. Conversation partners can also use strategies to change their own communication to support the communication of the person with a communication impairment. The conversation partner might be a spouse, a friend, an adult child or another healthcare professional, such as a nurse. Training the conversation partner is widely used as a treatment tool, especially for conversational partners of people with aphasia with programmes such as the SPPARRC (Supporting Partners of People with Aphasia in Relationships and Conversation) (Lock et al., 2008).

As mentioned in Chapter 3, an intervention by Williams et al. (2005) to help nursing staff be aware of their use of elderspeak helped to reduce the incidence of elderspeak use, leading to more effective and fulfilling communication interactions.

The use of video feedback and role play can help a conversation partner to work on aspects of their communication.

Outcomes

Outcomes of treatment need to provide a measure against the client's goals to evaluate whether these goals have been met. There are various formal outcome measures in use across services, and those chosen for a particular service will often gather data to show how the service is meeting organisational targets. These certainly have their place in terms of service provision but also need to be adaptable for client-centred goals. Most of the formal outcome measures will include measures of quality of life. For example, the widely used Therapy Outcome Measures (Enderby and John, 2015) has measurements that cover the domains of impairment, activity, participation and wellbeing.

Self-reported measures can also be used alongside more formal measures and are a good way of helping the client to see the change. Self-rating scales are a popular tool for this and can be easily replicated to be used in both baseline and outcome measurements. As well as the quantitative data, clinicians working with older people might find it beneficial to add flexibility into the outcome measures by recording some qualitative experiences or client stories. These are often useful to look back on when working with future clients or for students to look through. They are also an invaluable resource if a clinician is asked to give a presentation about their work to people who are not familiar with their service.

Follow-up

When a client has finished this episode of assessment or intervention, arrangements need to be made for follow-up. Follow-up of older patients is necessary to track their communication impairment. Other disorders associated with communication impairment are more likely to develop in older age, and these can be picked up at follow-up review. For example, a client presenting with what appears to be age-related word finding difficulties in the clinic might show significant deterioration of communication after a repeat of the baseline language screen at the follow-up review and, therefore, require further investigation.

Sometimes, a diagnosis is not fully known until it is seen how the symptoms develop with the passage of time. For instance, word finding difficulties can be an early symptom of dementia but might also be a simple age-related change. Voice changes can be the first symptom of a progressive neurological disorder or just a temporary impairment related to lifestyle factors such as poor voice care.

Follow-up time will vary according to the nature of impairment and the service provision. These appointments can be face to face or via telephone. However, a follow-up appointment is an ideal opportunity to repeat some of the assessment tasks in order to track symptoms.

If the symptoms are very mild or if the service is not set up to be able to offer follow-up appointments, the client and family can be educated in what symptoms to watch out for (e.g. significant deterioration of symptoms, memory problems and swallowing problems).

Case examples

Case example 1

William, known as Bill, is an 88-year-old who was referred to speech and language therapy by his doctor after experiencing episodes of word finding difficulty. As well as referral to SLT, his doctor arranged for investigations to rule out a stroke. These came back clear with no definitive evidence of stroke.

Case history: Bill and his family have noticed a gradual onset to his episodes of word finding difficulty. They are most noticeable during telephone calls. Bill lives alone following a divorce many years ago and has two children and three grandchildren. He used to enjoy trips out with his walking group, but this has recently been difficult due to a decline in physical health. He is interested in local history. He is independent with all activities of daily living and has no other medical symptoms apart from hypertension, which is managed with medication. He has some hearing loss and wears bilateral hearing aids.

Screening assessment: The screening test indicated no overall concern regarding speech or language apart from one episode of word finding difficulty.

Formal assessment: Picture-naming assessments indicated word finding difficulty on around one-third of the pictures. He responded well to phonological cueing (giving the first sound or first two sounds to prompt retrieval of the word).

Informal assessment: Informal assessment comprised description of a picture and general conversation. Bill appeared hesitant to begin with in the picture description task, and some episodes of word finding difficulty were noted. He was able to retrieve the correct word after a few attempts or with phonological cueing. In general conversation, Bill's language was fluent, with only a few episodes of word finding difficulty noted towards the end of the session. A word finding episode was signalled by a pause, hesitant speech, occasional repetition of the first sound and observed frustration in his facial expressions.

Other observations: Bill appeared to find the episodes of word finding difficulty frustrating and appeared to be very aware of them. He reports that this has made him reluctant to speak with people other than his family. The SLT felt that his word finding difficulties at this stage appeared to be consistent with his age.

Joint goal setting:

- To learn and practise strategies to facilitate word finding.
- To keep a log of when word finding difficulties are most evident.
- To use word finding strategies with family in conversation.
- To seek out a suitable social activity.
- To practise word finding strategies when talking with new people.

Intervention: Intervention consisted of three 30-minute sessions over the course of six weeks. Strategies for word finding were discussed with Bill. These included giving himself time, becoming comfortable with explaining what was happening when a word finding difficulty occurred and talking around the word or trying to retrieve the first sound of the word to prompt retrieval of the word. He practised these with picture and object naming in the clinic. He was also prompted to use them when word finding difficulty occurred in conversation with the SLT or accompanying family member.

Keeping a log of when his word finding difficulties are most evident indicated that they tend to occur most frequently when he is talking on the phone in the evenings and so likely to be linked with tiredness.

Follow-up: Bill was seen in the clinic again after three months. His family had moved telephone calls to the daytime, which had helped his conversation. He is attending a local social coffee-and-chat group, which he reports has improved his confidence. Assessments were repeated and indicated lower scores than previously, and the screening test indicated some difficulty following two-part instructions. His family also report some short-term memory loss. It was agreed that he would be referred back to his doctor with a request for an assessment of cognition and that he would be reviewed by SLT again in two months for further assessment and advice.

Case example 2

Doris is an 85-year-old who was referred to speech and language therapy by her doctor after her family noticed frequent episodes of word finding difficulty.

Case history: Doris lives on her own after her husband died two years ago. She has three children and five grandchildren. She used to enjoy going to meet her friends in the local coffee shop but has been more reluctant to do this recently. She still visits the local shop every day. She reports that she does not like talking much, gets tired easily and feels lonely. She takes medication for gastro-oesophageal reflux and for hypertension. She has some hearing loss and wears bilateral hearing aids.

Screening assessment: There were no overall concerns about speech or language apart from word finding difficulties. She took a little time to respond to questions, but this was felt to be within the limits of normal processing speed.

Formal assessment: In picture-naming tasks, episodes of word finding difficulty were noted on several of the pictures. Difficulty was indicated by hesitant speech and phrases, such as 'I know what it is'.

Informal assessment: In picture description and conversation, word retrieval episodes were less evident in general conversation. However, Doris was not forthcoming with conversation, and it was difficult to obtain a good language sample. She was tearful at times.

Other observations: SLT noticed that Doris was tearful and reluctant to engage in conversation and noticed a decline in her recent social activities. When asked about her mood, she admitted she was feeling low and missing her husband.

Joint goal setting: Doris felt that her speech was not her main priority at the moment. Following discussion, the following goals were identified:

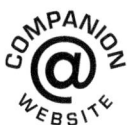

- SLT to contact Doris' doctor to request an assessment of her mood.
- Doris and her family to keep a log of when word finding difficulties are more evident.
- SLT to make a referral to the befriending service organised by a local charity.

Follow-up: Doris was seen back in the clinic after three months. After discussion with her doctor and an assessment of her mental health, she had decided to trial some medication for her low mood and was signposted to a bereavement charity for support. She felt her mood had improved. She had several telephone conversations with a volunteer from the befriending service and had started to meet her friends again for coffee. Her word finding difficulties were still evident, and she had found that these occurred more when she was tired or had not talked with anyone for a couple of days. She felt she was now able to engage in a few sessions of speech and language therapy to work on strategies, and she was put on the waiting list for this.

Resources

- Communication symptoms checklist
- Communication case history proforma
- Strategies to improve processing of spoken information
- Strategies to improve word finding difficulties
- Voice care advice for older people

Communication symptoms checklist

Before you attend your speech and language therapy appointment, please can you monitor your communication over a week or so, and you or a close relative or friend fill in this checklist of symptoms (see Table 5.2). The term 'communication' describes any speech or language, spoken or written. Filling in this checklist will help your clinician to understand the areas of communication you are having difficulty with and to be able discuss these with you in more detail at your appointment.

Table 5.2 Communication symptoms checklist

Please tick the areas you have difficulty with.	
Hearing	
Understanding what people are saying to you	
Following conversations	
Processing information	
Articulating speech sounds	

(Continued)

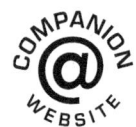

Table 5.2 (Continued)

Please tick the areas you have difficulty with.	
Knowing what to say but can't find the word	
Remembering names of people or objects	
Forming sentences	
Remembering the topic of conversation	
Participating in conversation	
Reading	
Writing	

Please describe any other communication symptoms.

Is there any pattern to your symptoms that you have noticed (e.g. morning versus evening, presence of background noise etc.)?

Communication case history proforma

Table 5.3 Communication case history proforma

Name **DOB** **NHS no**
Reason for referral
Past medical history
Medication / side effects
Smoking status
Alcohol intake
Recent medical investigations

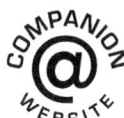

Visual/hearing impairment
Sleeping habits / energy levels (e.g. average sleep time, level of tiredness after daily activities and any recent changes)
Means of communication in an emergency situation
Client account of communication impairment
Nature of onset of impairment (e.g. gradual, occasional or chronic, and speed of deterioration)
Pre-impairment communication style (e.g. introvert/extravert, talkative, social or preferred own company)
Impact of communication impairment on current quality of life
Family/social networks
Impact of communication impairment on mood
Expectations of appointment / patient goals around communication

Strategies to improve processing of spoken information

The speed of hearing and understanding what other people are saying is known as processing speed, and this tends to slow down as we get older. This is a naturally occurring process but can occur with varying degrees of severity. Hearing impairment can be a complicating factor.

Here are some strategies to help with processing of spoken information:

- Reduce background noise or distractions where possible.
- Have your hearing checked.

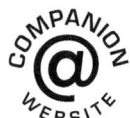

- Wear hearing aids if you need them.
- Consider that tiredness can affect processing speed. Try to get enough rest and avoid important conversations if you are feeling tired.
- Know that stress can affect processing speed, as the brain is distracted by competing demands.
- Ask people to give you one piece of information at a time and give you time to process what they have said.
- Ask people to speak more slowly if this helps.

If you notice any other symptoms, such as not understanding what has been said even when it is processed or having any memory difficulties, please contact your doctor.

Strategies to improve word finding difficulties

It is very common to have episodes where you know what you want to say but it seems that the right word can't find the way from your brain to your mouth. This is also called tip-of-the-tongue phenomenon and can be frustrating. These episodes can become more frequent in older age. Here are some strategies that can help with these episodes of word finding difficulty:

- Keep a physical or mental note of when the word finding difficulties occur in order to see whether there is any pattern (e.g. type of activity, time of day and type of conversation).
- Consider that tiredness can cause more frequent episodes of word finding difficulty. Try to get enough rest and avoid important conversations or speaking on the telephone where possible when you are feeling tired.
- Know that feeling anxious or tense can contribute to word finding difficulty, especially if the anxiety is around speaking. Try to remember that word finding difficulty is normal in older age, and notice that other people also have hesitant speech.
- Try to reduce distractions, such as having background noise, speaking with lots of people at once or multitasking, as these can make word finding difficulties worse.
- Consider that some people find it frustrating when other people fill in the words for them when they are struggling to find the word. Talk to people you are comfortable with and tell them whether you prefer them to fill in the word for you or if you would like to try to find it on your own.
- Try to think of the first sound or letter of the word, or think of how long the word is. This can sometimes prompt a quicker retrieval of the word.

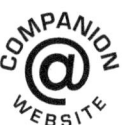

- Try to describe features of what the word means (e.g. it's an animal with four legs). This can prompt retrieval of the word and also gives other people a clue to what you are trying to say.
- Think of a different word that could be used to say the same thing. Again, this can sometimes prompt the actual word to appear.
- Take a break, if possible, or talk about something else and come back to it later. Sometimes, trying too hard can make it harder for the word to appear.

If your word finding difficulties are getting more frequent or if you experience any other symptoms, such as difficulty understanding what is being said and emotional, memory or swallowing problems, please contact your doctor.

Voice care advice for older people

This is adapted from Martin (2021) *Working with Voice Disorders: Theory and Practice, 3rd edition*.

Some voice changes are common in older people. The vocal cords become drier, and there might be less breath support to project the voice. These changes are usually gradual and subtle. Here is some advice to help take care of your voice and reduce the effects of age-related changes:

- Try not to raise your voice unnecessarily to talk above loud background noise (e.g. at loud social events).
- Avoid smoking. Speak to your doctor about support for smoking cessation if required.
- Limit alcohol intake as much as possible
- Avoid speaking on the telephone excessively.
- Avoid spicy foods and dairy products, which may affect your voice quality.
- Avoid eating a large meal before bed, as this can cause acid reflux, which can affect voice quality.
- Be aware that emotions can affect voice quality (e.g. tension, anxiety and depression can be reflected in the voice). Contact your doctor if you require support regarding your emotional wellbeing.
- Drink fluids (alcohol not included) regularly to avoid a dry throat affecting voice quality.
- Avoid dry atmospheres.
- Rest your voice if it is hoarse. Do not whisper or try to speak through the hoarseness.

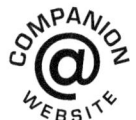

If you notice persistent or deteriorating voice change or accompanying symptoms, such as swallowing problems, please contact your doctor for further investigation.

References

Enderby, P and John, A (2015) *Therapy Outcome Measures for Rehabilitation Professionals*. 3rd Edition. J & R Press Ltd.

Lock, S, Wilkinson, R and Bryan, K (2008) *Supporting Partners of People with Aphasia in Relationships and Conversation*. Routledge.

Williams, K, Kemper, S and Hummert ML (2005) Enhancing communication with older adults: Overcoming elderspeak. *Journal of Psychosocial Nursing and Mental Health Services*. 43 (5): 12-16.

EATING, DRINKING AND SWALLOWING IN THE CONTEXT OF OLDER AGE

DOI: 10.4324/9781003058090-7

Introduction

The process of eating, drinking and swallowing forms a major part of our day-to-day lives. The process is not just physical; it is intrinsically linked with psychological, cultural and social factors. Of primary significance, eating and drinking are life sustaining functions, as our bodies require sufficient nutrition and hydration to remain alive. Not having optimal nutrition or hydration affects all the systems of the body, leading to increased vulnerability to illness and injury, and reduced recovery rates.

Social and cultural values are interwoven in the preparation of food and drink, and the act of eating and drinking together provides an opportunity to connect with other people. Certain foods might be selected depending on religious beliefs. There is also a strong emotional element to eating and drinking, with food and drink being central to the marking of both joyful occasions, such as a wedding celebration or a more sombre occasion, such as a funeral. Individual food and drink choices might evoke nostalgia or memories triggered by their sight, smell and taste.

The physiological process of swallowing is complex, requiring the delicate coordination of neuromuscular and sensory pathways to ensure a timely and safe passage of food and drink from the mouth to the stomach. This process is often described in phases: pre-oral, oral preparatory and oral, pharyngeal and oesophageal phases. Each phase will be discussed in more detail in the second section of this chapter, alongside a comparison of the effect of the ageing process on each phase.

The act of eating, drinking and swallowing becomes different as our bodies age. As with other age-related changes, this process also alters gradually in most healthy older people and with varying severity depending on the underlying reserve of the older person. The delicate process of swallowing is easily interfered with, and any changes to eating, drinking and swallowing can lead to a significant impact on an older person's quality of life. It appears that there is little awareness in the general public of the changes to eating, drinking and swallowing in older age, and the impact of these on an individual and the people close to them.

Swallowing impairments, commonly termed 'dysphagia', are a common symptom of many diseases that are more prevalent in the older population. Dysphagia itself is so common amongst the older population in relation to sarcopenia, frailty and other disorders that consideration has been given as to whether it should be included as a geriatric syndrome alongside other geriatric syndromes, such as incontinence or frailty (Baijens et al., 2016). Geriatric syndromes have been defined as conditions that are prevalent in older age, associated with multiple comorbidities and poor outcomes but that are multifactorial and do not necessarily fit a particular disease category (Baijens et al., 2016).

Age-related swallowing changes are sometimes termed as 'presbyphagia', which sets it apart from disease-related dysphagia. However, given the increased prevalence of disease-related dysphagia in older age, both presbyphagia and disease-related dysphagia will co-occur in many older adults. For the purpose of clarity in this book, age-related swallowing changes will be referred to as age-related swallowing changes or impairment, with pathological swallowing impairments referred to as dysphagia.

This chapter is divided into sections. The following section will explore general potential age-related changes to the eating, drinking and swallowing process, and the impact of these. The next section provides more detail about the phases of the swallow in healthy adults and the comparison with healthy older adults to reflect what are thought to be normal age-related changes to each phase. The final sections discuss what would be considered to be atypical features of an older person's swallowing, the effect of overall loss of reserve on the swallowing mechanism and disease-related dysphagia, and also the implications of swallowing impairment in older age.

General changes to the eating and drinking process in older adults

Lifestyle changes in older age are linked with changes to eating and drinking habits. This will look different for each older person but is related to the significance of the lifestyle change and overall health and wellbeing. For example, for some older people, retirement from working life can release more time to cook and prepare food, but for others, the lack of routine and structure in the day could make it more difficult to plan meals. The loss of a significant other is likely to lead to a change in cooking and eating habits as well as appetite changes associated with grief and loss. Some older people will stick with their longstanding food preferences or become more limited in what they eat, whereas others might become more adventurous and enjoy trying different foods. If an older person has a stay in a hospital or moves to a care home, their eating and drinking habits might become more institutionalised, with the possibility of fewer choices and stricter mealtimes, which might not align with their natural eating style.

Appetite changes are common in older people. Dry mouth, altered taste and dental changes can lead to eating and drinking becoming both less desirable and more uncomfortable, which negatively impacts on food intake. These will be described in more detail later in the chapter.

Physiological and metabolic changes to the ageing body also contribute. The stomach empties its contents more slowly (Firth and Prather, 2002), leading to increased digestive discomfort and longer feeling of fullness. Delayed gastric emptying can also lead to pressure on the lower oesophageal sphincter, thereby increasing the risk of gastro-oesophageal reflux (Fass et al., 2009). Hormonal changes or the body's responses to hormones, such as cholecystokinin, leptin and testosterone, can negatively impact the desire to eat, with subsequently reduced oral intake (Cichero, 2018).

The consequences of poor eating choices and undernourishment are significant with inadequate nutrition, one of the prognostic indicators for reduced cognitive and physical reserve in later life (see Chapter 2).

Some older people do not drink enough fluids. This may be because they do not realise the importance of regular fluid intake or do not have the same thirst signals. Cognitive impairment can cause forgetfulness around drinking. Decreased fluid intake can lead to complications, such as dehydration and increased risk of urinary tract infections, which can have serious consequences for older people, such as sepsis (Gharbi et al, 2019), delirium and increased hospitalisation.

Age-related postural changes may have an influence on swallowing ability. Kyphosis of the spine (curvature of the thoracic section of the spine) occurs with age to varying degrees (Katzman et al., 2010). For those older people with a more significant kyphosis, the ability to maintain a good upright posture to facilitate the timely and safe passage of food or drink into the stomach might be restricted.

Anecdotally, older people often report difficulty swallowing tablets. In their 2016 systematic review, McGillicuddy, Crean and Sahm found limited evidence supporting this, although the studies were restricted to older people living in their own homes. Nevertheless, given the importance of medications and the fact that older people tend to take multiple medications, these reports of difficulty swallowing tablets need to be taken seriously. Advice can be sought from the pharmacist or doctor on different formulations or consistencies of medications that can be offered. The client should be discouraged to make any modifications to the medication themselves in the absence of professional advice, as this can have implications for effectiveness and safety.

Effect of age on the phases of swallowing

The typical, normal swallow is described here in terms of phases of swallowing, although it is acknowledged that the phases can overlap. For example, it is known that some of the food bolus can slip into the pharynx during the oral stages in healthy individuals (Matsuo and Palmer, 2009), creating a blur between the oral and pharyngeal stages. The swallowing process is an intricate and complicated process involving coordination of nerves, muscles and structures (see Diagram 6.1). For the purposes of this chapter, however, the typical phases of swallowing are discussed in broad terms to allow for a later comparison between both the normal and the ageing swallow (see Table 6.1).

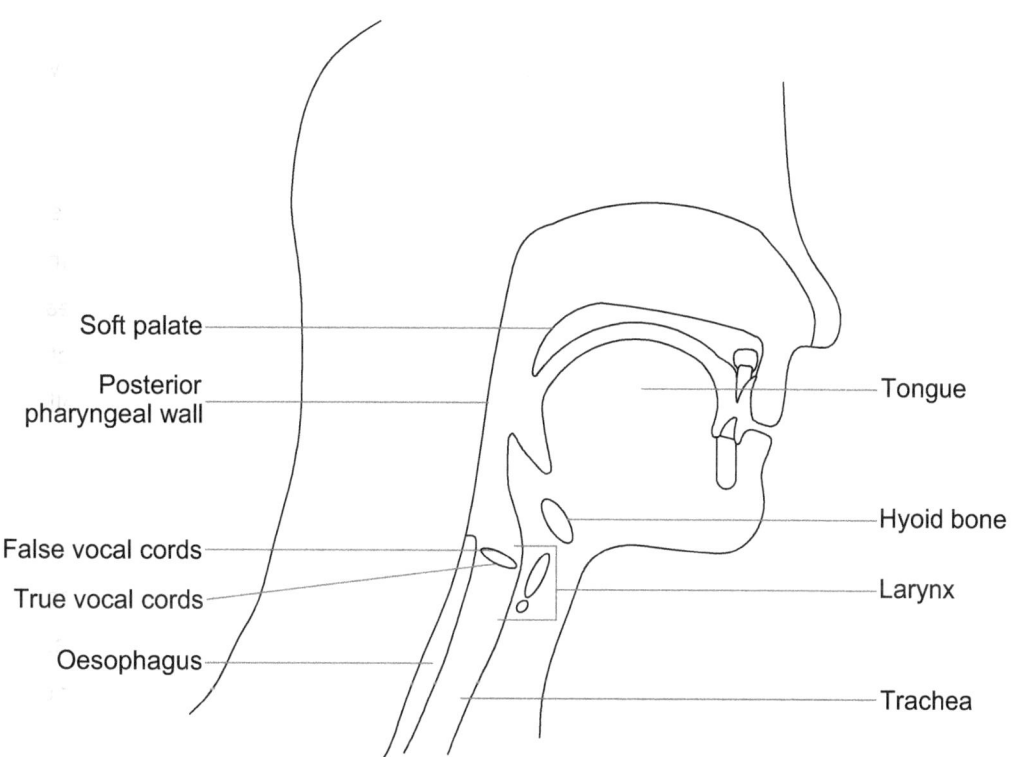

Diagram 6.1 *A midsagittal aspect of the head and neck, which illustrates some of the structures involved in the phases of swallowing*

The pre-oral phase

The pre-oral phase of swallowing can be viewed as a setting of the scene phase. It is largely a sensory phase, involving, for example, the visual stimuli of food or drink, the sounds of the cutlery and the smell of the food. It also includes the motor mechanisms of bringing food or drink to the open mouth. This phase should not be overlooked, as the sum of the sensory pre-oral experience creates the foundations of an effective swallow. It has been shown that the visual stimuli of food can start to excite the neurophysiological process of swallowing (Steele et al., 2010), and olfactory stimuli increases salivation in preparation for breaking down the bolus of food to swallow (Ebihara et al., 2006). The established motor patterns for bringing the bolus to the mouth via a cup, fingers or utensils also provide motor and sensory stimuli to the brain to prepare for the process of swallowing.

Effects of normal ageing at the pre-oral phase include a decline in the olfactory system and increase in the difficulty of discriminating between smells (Boyce et al., 2006). This can lead to a sensory impairment in the smelling of food or drink, which might lead to a reduction in the body's preparation for swallowing and a decrease in the production of saliva that is later required to assist with chewing and transferring a bolus of food through the mouth. Visual impairments can affect someone's ability to see or distinguish the food on their plate.

Some older adults will be entrenched in the routine of eating and drinking at similar times, eating and drinking the same items, and using the same equipment, so these cues can help to trigger an efficient swallow process. Interruptions to this pattern have the potential to disrupt these cues. This is the case if older people become less able to feed themselves as they are not so engaged in the process of the pre-oral phase or if there are fundamental changes to the eating or drinking environment or routine, such as with an admission to the hospital. That said, some older people with cognitive impairment or significantly reduced sensory signals might benefit from increased sensory cueing (see Chapter 7).

Oral preparatory and oral phases

The oral preparatory phase of the swallow starts as the bolus of food or fluid moves through the open lips. A solid bolus is masticated in order to break it down sufficiently for safe swallowing. This occurs with the help of saliva to moisten and soften the bolus, rotary jaw actions moving the teeth to break the bolus down and tongue movements to move the bolus in between the teeth. For both fluid and solids, adequate tone in the lips prevents the bolus from escaping anteriorly out of the mouth and tone in the cheek muscles limit food or fluid falling into the lateral sulci between the lower gums and inside cheek. Sensation within the oral cavity helps to locate the bolus and, combined with taste sensation, provides sensory signals ready for the next phases of swallowing.

The oral phase follows once the bolus is sufficiently broken down and is in a relatively cohesive form. The blade of the tongue begins to push the bolus up against the hard palate and backwards towards the soft palate and back of the oral cavity in preparation for the pharyngeal phase of the swallow. A moist mouth with adequate saliva also aids this transfer. The tongue remains high as the bolus is moved towards the back of the mouth to reduce movement of the bolus back to the front of the mouth. However, there may be some movement back and forth.

For a liquid bolus, the tongue can form a channel in the centre to help transport the liquid to the back of the mouth.

Age-related changes in these phases include the following:

Dentition

It is not unusual to lose teeth in older age, and this will affect the ability to chew and bite. Denture wearing may affect the ability to chew some foods effectively, and there is evidence that people who wear them often naturally start to avoid foods that are difficult to bite into (Abdul Razak et al., 2014). Dentures can become loose with weight loss or changes to the oro-facial musculature, which also affects the ability to chew efficiently.

Oral health

The oral health of older people can be affected by altered saliva production and subsequent dry mouth. This occurs as a natural part of the ageing process to varying degrees but can be exacerbated by the side effects of medication or residual consequences of treatment, such as radiotherapy. In the oral preparatory stage, reduced saliva can limit the ability to break down a specially dry foodstuff into a cohesive bolus ready for swallowing and subsequently leave some food remaining in the mouth. Dry mouth and residue of food in the oral cavity can also result in the build-up of bacteria on the tongue and the other mucous membranes in the mouth, leading to increased risk of infection, altered taste and discomfort when eating and drinking. Abdul Razak et al. (2014) report that periodontal disease is one of the most prevalent disorders in older age.

Taste sensation

The sensation of taste in older age can change as a direct result of age-related change to the olfactory system with the interplay of the sensations of smell and taste. Taste changes can be related to density of taste buds. Toffanello et al. (2013) report that age-related taste changes are not geographically equal in terms of density of taste buds on the tongue, with older people tending to retain sensation for sweeter tastes but experiencing a decline in the detection of sour, bitter and salty tastes.

Tongue muscles

Fujishima et al. (2019) and Ney et al. (2009) both report weakness in the tongue due to naturally occurring sarcopenia in healthy older age. Namasivayam et al. (2018) found that tongue movements can become slower and more variable in older age. Ney et al. (2009) conclude that although there is sarcopenia of the tongue muscles in older age, this should not prevent healthy older adults from achieving an effective swallow.

Older people masticate their food for longer, which has been found to be linked both with natural age-related change and reduced dentition (Kohyama et al., 2003). Cichero (2018) stated that chewing function remains unchanged, but age-related sarcopenia and reduced dentition can lead to altered food choices and reduced chewing efficiency.

Logemann (2014) observes that older people are more likely to use a dipper technique to establish bolus transfer in the oral phase of swallowing. This involves the tongue tip sliding forwards to pick up the bolus on to the tongue, as opposed to the tipper technique where the bolus is placed on the top of the tongue directly. She concludes that the dipper initiation of the oral stage can prolong posterior oral transfer of the bolus in older people.

Pharyngeal phase

The pharyngeal phase of swallowing is an involuntary phase. It begins the as the bolus passes through the faucial pillars the back of the oral cavity, although the pharyngeal swallow is not necessarily initiated at this point.

Anticipatory sensory stimulation in preparation for this phase of the swallow is also accumulated from the pre-oral and oral stages. The actual position of the bolus of food or fluid at the time of initiation of the pharyngeal swallow varies from person to person, with studies of healthy individuals revealing that food or fluid can enter the top of the pharynx into the vallecular space before the swallow is initiated (Matsuo and Palmer, 2009).

During the pharyngeal phase, the soft palate is elevated to close off the nasopharynx to prevent escape of the bolus through the nasal passages. The base of tongue pushes against the posterior pharyngeal wall to create pressure to help the bolus propel through the pharynx.

The critical objective of this phase is to get the bolus through the pharynx into the oesophagus without it or parts of it entering the airway and potentially being aspirated (aspiration refers to the bolus passing below the level of the vocal cords and entering the lungs). In order to achieve maximum closure of the airway, the hyoid bone and larynx are pulled upwards and forwards, which leads to deflection of the epiglottis over the laryngeal vestibule; the vocal cords close over the glottis, and closure of the false vocal cords superior to the vocal cords provides additional protection.

The bolus moves through the pharynx with the help of gravity, pressure generation from the base of tongue pushing against the posterior pharyngeal wall and constriction of the pharyngeal muscles. The upper oesophageal sphincter is pulled open as a result of the movement of the larynx and the sensory signal of the bolus head against the sphincter muscle. In total, this pharyngeal phase is thought to last around one second (Matsuo and Palmer, 2009).

Typical ageing influences the pharyngeal stage of the swallow in various ways. Reduced tongue pressure can affect the pressure generated by the base of tongue pushing against the posterior pharyngeal wall and, combined with reduced strength of the pharyngeal constrictor muscles, can lead to increased residue of the bolus in the pharynx post swallow (Fujishima et al., 2019).

A review into the timing of the swallow in older people carried out by Namasivayam et al. (2018) concluded that there is a longer reaction time between the bolus entering the pharynx and the onset of hyoid-laryngeal movement. Ney et al. (2009) agree that there is slower initiation of pharyngeal and laryngeal movement due to reduced strength or slower innervation of the suprahyoid muscle. Ney et al. (2009) also report that laryngeal penetration (where the bolus enters the larynx but does not pass below the vocal cords) occurs more frequently and to a greater depth with increasing age. Bowing of the vocal cords can arise in older age due to weakness or atrophy in either or both vocal cords. Depending on the severity of the bowing, it can lead to incomplete glottal closure, which can increase the risk of aspiration.

Shaker (Shaker et al, 2003) tested glottal closure reflex using rapid pulse injections of water and found that it took a larger volume of water to stimulate this reflex in older subjects. This suggests reduced sensory recognition and increased need to optimise the sensory signals in preparation for swallowing.

Namasivayam et al. (2018) report a longer duration of upper oesophageal sphincter opening in older adults, with a slower return to its resting closed position. This is likely to increase the risk of reflux or regurgitation, particularly if a person reclines after mealtimes.

Oesophageal phase

The oesophageal phase of swallowing commences at the level of the upper oesophageal sphincter as it opens to allow the bolus to pass into the oesophagus. Peristaltic movement of the oesophageal muscles move the bolus along to the lower oesophageal sphincter at the gastro-oesophageal junction, which opens to allow the bolus to move into the stomach.

There has been much discussion and research into the effects of ageing on the oesophageal phase of swallowing. Robbins et al. (2006) suggest findings of studies focusing on age-related changes can be contradictory and difficult to compare due to the variety of tools used to gather the data. Besanko et al. (2014) report that there is reduced relaxation of the lower oesophageal sphincter in older adults, which can lead to increased residue in the oesophagus.

Gregerson et al. (2008) found that oesophageal peristalsis starts to reduce after the age of 40. However, Robson et al. (2003) report no significant age differences either in relaxation of the lower oesophageal sphincter or in peristaltic movement.

Summary of typical changes to the phases of swallowing in older age

The overall picture of the ageing swallow is one of slower sensory response and slower and weaker muscular movements (sarcopenia) occurring alongside behavioural and lifestyle changes. The extent to which the ageing process affects the swallow may be influenced by the factors that predict the speed of age-related change, such as overall fitness and strength, cognition, nutrition and genetic predisposition.

Table 6.1 Summary of the ageing effects on the process of swallowing

Pre-oral phase	Less acute sense of smell
	Visual changes
	More sensitive to changes in environmental or physical cues
Oral preparatory phase	Altered taste sensation; may develop more of a preference towards sweeter tastes
	Deterioration of dentition
	Increased risk of periodontal disease and poor oral hygiene
	Slower tongue movements
	Reduced tongue strength
Oral phase	Slower oral transfer of the bolus
	Reduced tongue strength and slower tongue movements

Pharyngeal phase	Slower initiation of pharyngeal swallow
	Weaker tongue affecting pressure generation for propulsion of bolus
	Weaker pharyngeal constriction
	Increased bolus residue in pharynx
	Reduced sensory awareness
	Increased frequency and depth of laryngeal penetration of bolus
	Incomplete glottal closure
	Longer duration of upper oesophageal sphincter opening
Oesophageal phase	Contradictory findings
	Reduced peristaltic wave
	Reduced relaxation of lower oesophageal sphincter

Atypical features of age-related swallowing changes and disease-related dysphagia

Dysphagia as a response to acute illness, infection or injury in older adults

The effect of ageing on the swallowing process means that there is a loss of available reserve to protect the safety of the swallow if the body is exposed to further stressors. If the body is under stress and busy fighting an infection or recovering from illness, there are fewer resources available to ensure a smooth and safe swallowing process. The just about safe and functional elderly swallow can easily tip into a disordered swallow (dysphagia) that is more vulnerable to frequent aspiration events or choking. Age-related changes, such as the slowing down of the swallow process, the weakness of the tongue muscles or the slower closure of the airway, will be more pronounced.

The impact of the loss of swallow reserve is more pronounced in some older people than others in line with the spectrum of severity of age-related change. Loss of reserve can also be more prevalent amongst older people with a history of stroke, which may have caused a residual swallow weakness, making it more vulnerable to age-related change.

Infections such as urinary tract infections (UTI) and trauma such as hip fractures are common amongst older people. The reduced reserve and resilience of an ageing swallow described earlier explain why some older people who are exposed to an infection or other trauma suddenly seem to start coughing when swallowing or displaying other symptoms of dysphagia when there is no apparent history of any disease-causing dysphagia.

A dysphagia as a result of an acute infection or trauma is sometimes referred to as a 'decompensated swallow'. One would expect that this type of dysphagia would improve as the body recovers, and it is certainly the case that the swallow does improve in such circumstances. That said, there are contributing factors to how much the swallow is able to improve, and these include baseline health and the ability to access good nutrition, hydration and mobilisation during the recovery period (Fujishima et al., 2019). Repeated infections and ongoing age-related sarcopenia or frailty may lead to a scenario in which the swallow cannot recover to or near to its original state.

Frailty

Age-related swallowing impairment and dysphagia are both a precursor to and a consequence of frailty in older people. Cichero (2018) found that normal age-related changes to the eating, drinking and swallowing process predispose an older person to developing frailty. There can be a downward spiral in which avoiding difficult foods and altered appetite lead to nutritional deficiency and weight loss, which exacerbates frailty and, in turn, leads to a more significant dysphagia (Fujishima et al., 2019).

The effect of frailty on the eating, drinking and swallowing process is similar to that of age-related sarcopenia, but frailty is associated with a more pervasive, chronic weakness with significant loss of reserve. Frailty will lead to the swallow becoming less safe more quickly and more severely, even with more seemingly mild infection or trauma, and recovery will be significantly limited. Rofes et al. (2010) studied the swallowing process in frail elderly people using videofluoroscopy. They found increased oro-pharyngeal residue associated with impaired tongue propulsion. There was also reduced hyoid movement and slower closure of the laryngeal vestibule, leading to reduced airway protection. Aspiration occurred in 17% of the participants, and there were higher mortality rates at one year post study in frail elderly people with dysphagia compared to those with a healthy swallow.

Dysphagia as a symptom of a disease

Dysphagia is a common symptom of many of the diseases associated with increased prevalence in older age. A number of these diseases are listed in Table 6.2, although this is not an exhaustive list. Each one will affect the swallow in different ways, and there is not scope within this book to discuss the effects of each separately. However, for the purposes of this book, it is important for the reader to understand that alongside the swallowing symptoms related to each disease, there will be co-occurring age-related changes, and

Table 6.2 A list of some of the diseases in which dysphagia presents as a common symptom

Neurological	Stroke
	Head injury
	Progressive neurological disease (e.g. Parkinson's, motor neurone disease and cortico-basal degeneration)
	Dementia
	Delirium
	Brain tumour
Respiratory	Chronic obstructive pulmonary disease (COPD)
	Bronchiectasis
Structural	Pharyngeal pouch
	Severe kyphosis
	Osteophytes
	Post-surgical or radiological changes
Cancer	Head and neck cancers
	Oesophageal cancer
	Primary or metastatic brain tumours
	Lymphoma
	Lung cancer
Other oesophageal	Barrett's oesophagus
	Gastro-oesophageal reflux
	Hiatus hernia
	Achalasia

these need to be accounted for. For example, if a person has a stroke, one would expect some recovery of swallowing with rehabilitation therapy, but an older person's swallow would not rehabilitate to the same level as a younger person's swallow because of underlying age-related change.

Implications of swallowing changes and dysphagia in older age

The implications of restricted food choices and poor nutritional balance have already been mentioned in association with exacerbation of sarcopenia and decline into frailty. Any kind of swallowing difficulty has the potential to impact on a person's quality of life. Having to restrict food choices or experiencing distressing symptoms when eating and drinking can have a significant impact on a person's psychological health. Two of the more severe consequences of dysphagia are aspiration pneumonia and choking.

Aspiration, chest infections and aspiration pneumonia

As mentioned in the second section of the chapter, aspiration is when a material, such as food, liquid, secretions or gastric material, enters into the laryngeal vestibule and travels below the level of the vocal cords towards the lungs. This differs from laryngeal penetration, which is when material enters the laryngeal vestibule but not below the vocal cords. If the material reaches the vocal cords or passes near to them, a cough reflex is normally initiated to aid expulsion of it from the larynx back into the pharyngeal space. Aspiration can occur when a cough is not sufficient to clear the material from the airway or if a cough is not initiated (known as silent aspiration) and the material falls or drips below the vocal cords as they reopen following a swallow. It can also occur before or during a swallow if the airway is not closed off in a timely way or if it is not closed tightly enough.

Aspiration can occur in a single event, such as the inhalation of a pill, or as frequent episodes. The term micro-aspiration relates to ongoing, frequent episodes of aspirating small amounts of material, such as secretions or food residue. If the lungs are unable to clear aspirated material with effective coughing, then it has the potential to inflame the lungs and cause chest infections or pneumonia.

As noted earlier in the chapter, healthy older people experience more frequent laryngeal penetration of the bolus, and this occurs to a greater depth within the laryngeal vestibule, putting them at more risk of aspiration. The cough that is required to clear the material in the laryngeal vestibule can be less efficient in older age. Cichero (2018) explains that although the cough reflex sensitivity appears to remain unchanged, there is a reduction in the perceived urge to cough amongst older people, and that this is more pronounced in those who have frailty. Yamanda et al. (2008) studied frail older people with a history of repeat aspiration pneumonia and found a severely diminished urge to cough even with the use of strong stimuli to try and elicit a response.

Ebihara et al. (2016) associate micro-aspiration with chronic inflammation of the lungs (pneumonitis) in frail elderly people. Komatsu et al. (2018) report that aspiration pneumonia itself increases sarcopenia in the respiratory and swallowing muscles, thereby reducing the prospects of a good recovery. Aspiration pneumonia is a major complication for older adults and is associated with more frequent hospitalisation and increased mortality (Lanspa et al., 2013).

Not all aspiration events lead to a chest infection or a pneumonia. In their iconic study, Langmore et al. (1998) researched risk factors associated with the development of aspiration pneumonia and found multiple predictors. These predictors are independent of whether the person has dysphagia. However, people with dysphagia will aspirate more frequently than

Eating, drinking and swallowing

Table 6.3   Risk factors for developing aspiration pneumonia

Main risk factors for developing aspiration pneumonia (Langmore et al., 1998)
Dependence for oral care
Decayed teeth
Multiple medications
Being fed via a tube
Dependence for feeding
Smoking
Multiple morbidities

those without dysphagia and, therefore, are more likely to develop aspiration pneumonia if they have one or more of these predictors alongside their dysphagia. These risk factors are summarised in Table 6.3.

It is of importance to acknowledge that many of these will disproportionately apply to older people, such as taking multiple medications, having poor dentition or having diagnosis of multiple illnesses.

Choking

Choking can be defined as a blockage of the airway due to an obstruction, such as a bolus of food or an object. This restricts the ability to breathe efficiently, and the outcome can be fatal.

Poor dentition or loose dentures affect the ability to chew a bolus of food to a sufficiently small size, resulting in the increased possibility of swallowing a large bolus of food, which could drop into and block the airway. Similarly, reduced oral control of a food bolus or delayed initiation of the swallow can cause the bolus of food to drop into the pharynx and into the unprotected airway before the swallow is initiated. Drowsiness or distractibility can also contribute to a choking risk.

Fatality rates from choking is higher in the category of older people than in any other age group, and there are strong correlations between choking and diagnoses of Parkinson's disease, dementia and pneumonitis (Kramarow et al., 2014).

Chapter summary

- Swallowing changes in normal older age can be characterised by slower and weaker muscle movements, and slower sensory response alongside behavioural and lifestyle changes.

- An infection such as a UTI or a trauma such as a hip fracture can cause an ageing swallow to become a disordered swallow with increased risk of aspiration. The swallow can recover somewhat with overall recovery from the infection or trauma.

- There is a cycle in which appetite changes and avoidance of some foods lead to weight loss and poor nutrition, which in turn leads to increased sarcopenia and risk of frailty and increased risk of developing dysphagia.

- Older people are at more risk of developing diseases for which dysphagia is a common symptom. These dysphagia symptoms will occur on the background of age-related change.

- Older people are at increased risk of aspiration pneumonia and choking.

References

Abdul Razak, P, Jose Richard, KM and Thankachan, RP (2014) Geriatric oral health: A review article. *Journal of International Oral Health, International Journal of Preventative and Community Dentistry.* 6: 110-116, November-December 6.

Baijens, LWJ et al. (2016) European society for swallowing disorders- European Union geriatric medicine society white paper: Oro-pharyngeal dysphagia as a geriatric syndrome. *Clinical Interventions in Aging.* 11: 1403-1428.

Besanko, LK et al. (2014) Changes in esophageal and lower esophageal sphincter motility with healthy aging. *Journal of Gastrointestinal and Liver Diseases.* 3: 243-248, September 23.

Boyce, JM and Shone, GR (2006) Effects of ageing on smell and taste. *Postgraduate Medical Journal.* 82 (966): 239-241.

Cichero, JAY (2018) Age-related changes to eating and drinking impact frailty: Aspiration, choking risk, modified food texture and autonomy of choice. *Geriatrics.* 3: 69.

Ebihara, S et al. (2016) Dysphagia, dystussia and aspiration pneumonia in elderly people. *Journal of Thoracic Disorders.* 3: 632-639, March 8.

Ebihara, T et al. (2006) A randomised control trial of olfactory stimulation using black pepper oil in older people with swallowing dysfunction. *Journal of American Geriatrics Society.* 54 (9): 1401-1406.

Fass, R, McCallum, RW and Parkman, HP (2009) Treatment challenges in the management of gastroparesis-related GERD. *Gastroenterology and Hepatology.* 10 (Suppl 18): 4-16, October 5.

Firth, M and Prather, CM (2002) Gastrointestinal mobility problems in the elderly patient. *Gastroenterology.* 122 (6): 1688-1700.

Fujishima, I et al. (2019) Sarcopenia and dysphagia: Position paper by four professional organisations. *Geriatrics and Gerontology International.* 19 (2).

Gharbi, M et al. (2019) Antibiotic Management of urinary tract infection in elderly patients in primary care and its association with bloodstream infections and all cause mortality: Population based cohort study. *British Medical Journal.* 364: 1525.

Gregerson, H, Pederson, J and Mohr Drewes, A (2008) Deterioration of muscle function in the human oesophagus with age. *Digestive Diseases and Sciences.* 53 (12): 3065-3070.

Katzman, W et al. (2010) Age related hyperkyphosis: Its causes, consequences and management. *Journal of Orthopaedic and Sports Physical Therapy.* 40 (6).

Kohyama, K, Mioche, L and Bourdio, P (2003) Influence of age and dental status on chewing behaviour studied by EMG recordings during consumption of various food samples. *Gerodontology.* 1 (20).

Komatsu, R et al. (2018) Aspiration pneumonia induces muscle atrophy in the respiratory, skeletal and swallowing systems. *Journal of Cachexia, Sarcopenia and Muscle.* 9: 643-653.

Kramarow, E, Warner, M and Chen, H (2014) Food related choking deaths among the elderly. *Injury Prevention*. 3: 200–203, June 20.

Langmore, SE et al. (1998) Predictors of aspiration pneumonia: How important is dysphagia? *Dysphagia*. 13: 69–81.

Lanspa, MJ et al. (2013) Mortality, morbidity and disease severity of patients with aspiration pneumonia. *Journal of Hospital Medicine: An Official Publication of the Society of Hospital Medicine*. 2: 83–90, February 8.

Logemann, J (2014) Critical factors in the oral control needed for chewing and swallowing. *Journal of Texture Studies*. 45 (3): 173–179.

Matsuo, K and Palmer, J (2009) Anatomy and physiology of feeding and swallowing- normal and abnormal. *Physical Medicine and Rehabilitation Clinics of North America*. 4: 691–707, November 19.

McGillicuddy, A, Crean, AM and Sahm, LJ (2016) Older adults with difficulty swallowing oral medicines; a systematic review of the literature. *European Journal of Clinical Pharmacology*. 72: 141–151.

Namasivayam- MacDonald, AM, Barbon, CEA and Steele, CM (2018) A review of swallow timing in the elderly. *Physiology and Behaviour*. 184: 12–26, February 1.

Ney, DM et al. (2009) Senescent swallowing: Impact, strategies and interventions. *Nutrition in Clinical Practice*. 24 (3): 395–413, June–July.

Robbins, J, Duke Bridges, A and Taylor, A (2006) Oral, pharyngeal and esophageal motor function in ageing. *GI Motility Online*. doi 10.1038/gimo39. www.nature.com accessed 9/2/2021 at 13.23.

Robson, KM and Glick, ME (2003) Dysphagia and advancing age: are manometric abnormalities more common in older patients? Digestive Disease and Sciences Sept 48(9) 1709–12.

Rofes, L et al. (2010) Pathophysiology of oropharyngeal dysphagia in the frail elderly. *Neurogastroenterology and Motility*. 22 (8).

Shaker, R et al. (2003) Pharyngoglottal closure reflex: Characterisation in healthy young, elderly and dysphagic patients with predeglutitive aspiration. *Gerontology*. 49 (1).

Steele, CM and Millar, AJ (2010) Sensory input pathways and mechanisms in swallowing: A review. *Dysphagia*. 25 (4): 323–333.

Toffanello, ED et al. (2013) Taste loss in hospitalised elderly subjects. *Clinical Interventions in Ageing*. 8: 167–174.

Yamanda, S et al. (2008) Impaired urge to cough in elderly patients with aspiration pneumonia. *Cough*. 4: 11.

CLINICAL ASSESSMENT AND MANAGEMENT OF EATING, DRINKING AND SWALLOWING IN OLDER PEOPLE

DOI: 10.4324/9781003058090-8

Introduction

This chapter builds on the theoretical information of the previous chapter to show how this can be applied practically when working clinically with older people who have swallow impairments. It has a similar layout to Chapter 4, taking the client journey from pre-assessment and case history, assessment and interpretation, intervention, and outcomes. Speech and language therapists are the healthcare professionals with formal training to assess and manage swallow impairments, although older people are most likely to be referred to SLT from another health professional, such as a doctor, nurse or dietitian, who may have enquired about or noticed symptoms of swallow impairment.

The methods and tools SLTs use to assess and manage swallowing impairments in adults are ubiquitous across client groups. Therefore, the methods and interventions will be touched upon broadly and followed up with a focus on how these might apply to working with older clients.

Two case examples at the end of the chapter will highlight how this practical information can be applied in real-life clinical scenarios. Supporting clinical resources can also be found in the 'Resources' section of the chapter.

Clinical journey

Pre-assessment

Pending their initial assessment appointment, clients or carers can be invited to fill in some pre-assessment information. The pre-assessment profile in Chapter 2 will give the clinician an overview of the client's baseline health, risk factors for sarcopenia and subsequent swallow impairment.

Pertinent information can also be obtained by asking the client, carer or family member to fill in a diary of the swallow symptoms for one week before their appointment. Carrying out this activity can help the client or carers to pinpoint symptoms more specifically. Some older people might not have insight into their swallowing problem, or it may have been happening for so long that they have become used to the symptoms. Filling in a swallowing symptom diary before they attend the appointment can help them to become more aware. A proforma of a diary of symptoms can be found in the 'Resources' section (Table 7.6). The diary lists the various symptoms that present with swallow impairments to educate on what symptoms to look out for.

The information will assist the clinician to begin to see any patterns in the swallow symptoms that might signal an underlying cause.

Text message can be sent as a reminder to fill these in and bring to the appointment if the client has officially consented to this form of communication.

Case history

As we discussed in Chapter 4, the first step in meeting a new client is to gather information pertaining to the reason for referral to gain a context of the impairment both in a clinical context and in the wider context of its effect on the client's quality of life.

Taking a case history is an efficient method of collecting this information whilst also providing an opportunity for the client and clinician to start building their professional rapport.

In the 'Resources' section, there is a proforma of a case history for older clients presenting with swallowing concerns. The questions on the case history allow it to be used across various outpatient and inpatient settings, and are designed for the clinician to begin to identify the nature and context of the impairment. If the client has a communication impairment, pictures can be used to support the information-gathering process, or some information can be obtained via another healthcare professional or medical documentation.

Although the questions in this case history proforma are similar to the questions that would be addressed to any adult with symptoms of swallowing difficulty, the interpretation of the responses might be different. For example, an older person is more likely to have an underlying disease process, although this cannot be ruled out for younger adults. Weight loss and poor nutrition will be red flags for more severe age-related sarcopenia and risk of dysphagia and frailty.

The rationale behind some of the questions is discussed subsequently:

> *Nature of onset of impairment:* This helps the clinician to begin to formulate ideas about the cause of the swallow impairment. For example, a slow, gradual decline could be attributed to normal ageing. A faster, more severe decline with other symptoms, such as dysarthria, could indicate a progressive neurological disorder.
>
> *Oral hygiene:* Poor oral hygiene and poor dental health are linked with aspiration pneumonia (Langmore et al., 1998). Knowing about the client's oral health can provide an education opportunity to increase awareness of the link between poor

oral health and chest infections or pneumonia. The state of oral health might also influence the clinician's recommendations about how to manage the swallow impairment.

Smoking/alcohol status: Smoking and/or alcohol intake contribute to the risk of oral, pharyngeal and oesophageal cancers, which are more prevalent in older age categories, and dysphagia is a common symptom of these. Smoking also compromises respiratory health so can increase vulnerability to pneumonia as well as inhibit recovery.

Recent or recurring chest infections: Frequent chest infections can be a signal of chronic aspiration. If a person has a respiratory condition or if their chest is vulnerable to infection, they are more likely to develop a chest infection or pneumonia if they aspirate. Age-related sarcopenia can make the lungs more vulnerable to pneumonia and prolong recovery time.

Buying and preparation of food: The response to this question will help the clinician gain insight into the client's lifestyle and risk factors for dysphagia. A person who is living alone, does not cook and has little appetite will have a poorer prognosis than someone who cooks regularly or who has meals prepared for them and can eat a good, balanced diet. Any social or practical issues in this area will need to be addressed alongside the swallow impairment.

Weight management: Unintentional or unexplained weight loss can signal a variety of underlying conditions so always necessitates further investigation. Weight loss in older people is a risk factor for dysphagia as it leads to weakness and increased sarcopenia. Not being able to eat a balanced diet is also a risk factor for increased sarcopenia and frailty.

Impact of swallowing on quality of life: Individuals will differ as to how their swallowing symptoms are affecting their quality of life and in what ways. They may require some prompting questions, such as 'how have things changed since you started to experience swallowing difficulties?' and 'how does it make you feel?'.

Expectations of appointment / patient goals: The client may have already started to develop a theory on the nature of the swallowing difficulties or researched it on the internet. This can be a time to discuss these from the client's perspective and offer further explanation. It is useful to know what the client's current goals are so that these can be applied when the formal goal setting takes place following assessment.

Assessment

The next phase is to move on to more direct assessment of the swallow impairment. The results of this, combined with pre-assessment information and the case history, will provide a strong clinical picture of the swallow symptoms for the clinician to work from. Assessments can take place in a variety of settings, including outpatient clinics, inpatient wards, care homes or the client's own home. This is often due to convenience, time and circumstances rather than client choice, but it is useful to be aware of how presentation might be different in another environment, such as hospital versus home.

The range of swallow assessments that are routinely in use for adults with symptoms of swallow impairment are described in broad terms in Table 7.1.

All swallow assessments should include an evaluation of the client's oral and dental health.

Considerations for older clients

The type of assessment used will depend on the individual client, the reported concerns and service provision. The client's age should not preclude access to a particular assessment if that is felt to be the optimal assessment for the swallow symptoms.

Table 7.1   Types of swallow assessments

Type of assessment	Description
Swallow screen	Basic screen of swallow ability to identify overt symptoms of impairment. Usually carried out by a clinician other than SLT, such as nurses or doctors, but an SLT often trains them on the procedure of the screening. There are different swallow screens in use across different services. A commonly used one is the 3oz water swallow screen (DePippo et al., 1992). Swallow screens are versatile and can be used across different settings. The results of the screen will decide whether referral to SLT for a full swallow assessment is indicated. First line advice can be given following a swallow screen, and the results of the screen can help the SLT to triage patients based on the severity of their symptoms. The more subtle signs of swallow impairment, such as silent aspiration (when aspiration occurs without a cough response), are likely to be missed.
Mealtime observation	Observation of a client eating a meal is an informal assessment of the eating, drinking and swallowing process. A lot of information can be gleaned from these assessments, but they are unlikely to be as detailed as the bedside clinical swallow assessment or an instrumental assessment. Mealtime observations are easier to arrange in settings such as the client's home, hospital wards or nursing/care homes. Mealtime checklists can be used as a swallow screen, or SLTs can observe mealtimes as part of their detailed assessment. Symptoms of swallow impairment are noted during the observation. Mealtime observations are more natural than contrived clinical assessments and give the clinician insight into the real-life challenges that might occur with the swallow impairment. It also might feel more natural for the client to be eating in their own environment albeit being observed by a clinician.

Type of assessment	Description
Bedside clinical swallow assessment	These assessments are routinely carried out by speech and language therapists, with the aim of gathering information to form hypotheses on the nature and severity of the swallow impairment and the risk of aspiration pneumonia.
	Although commonly termed 'bedside assessment', they can be used in a variety of settings, such as hospital wards, outpatient clinics, nursing/care homes and client's own homes.
	Bedside assessments involve a cranial nerve assessment, trials of different bolus consistencies, tastes and sizes, and trials of different head postures or swallow techniques. The swallow is palpated digitally to estimate swallow timing and the level of hyo-laryngeal movement. SLTs use various other tools, such as cervical auscultation, pulse oximetry and cough sensitivity, and strength testing during these assessments.
	These assessments can give the clinician more detailed information about the client's swallowing ability than a mealtime assessment or screen. However, as the oral and pharyngeal stages of the swallowing cannot be actually visualised, the hypotheses are based on information from careful observation and interpretation of overt symptoms. Silent aspiration may well be missed.
Instrumental assessment	The two main instrumental assessments of swallowing used in speech and language therapy are videofluoroscopy (VF) and fibre-optic endoscopic evaluation of swallowing (FEES).
	Videofluoroscopic assessment of swallowing allows all the phases of the swallow to be viewed radiologically in real time and the effects of different bolus sizes and consistencies, head postures, or swallow strategies to be visualised. It can also detect silent aspiration and other impairments, such as pharyngeal pouch.
	FEES is also widely used. This enables visualisation of the part of the pharyngeal stage of swallowing. FEES allows observation of the effects of different bolus sizes and consistencies, head postures and swallows strategies in real time as well as identifying silent aspiration.
	Swallow impairments due to natural older age will be much more visible on these instrumental assessments, and so the clinician needs to be aware of what is in the normal range for an older person.

All clinicians will justify their assessment choice with rationale, and there may be specific justifications for older clients. For example, although a VF would give a more detailed and objective assessment of the phases of the swallow, the best swallow assessment for an older person with dementia in a care home who becomes easily disorientated might be a mealtime observation. Here, the clinician can observe the person's swallow in the real-life eating and drinking environment with little demand placed on the client, thereby reducing any distress. Strategies and advice can be given based on observation and monitoring.

People are more prone to fatigue with advancing age, and people with frailty especially might find that they become more tired over the course of the meal. In line with this, their swallowing will become less efficient and less safe over a meal. The best way to identify the effect of fatigue on an individual's swallow is to challenge the swallow with multiple oral trials during bedside assessment or to do an assessment over a mealtime when the client is likely to eat a larger amount.

An older person who has specific pharyngeal symptoms following a stroke would benefit most from a VF or FEES to identify the exact cause of the symptoms, reduce the risk of aspiration and assess suitability for specific rehabilitation techniques.

If an older adult is presenting with frequent chest infections of no clear cause it would be prudent to carry out a VF or FEES examination to rule out silent aspiration or micro-aspiration.

Quality of life assessment

Information on how the swallow impairment is affecting mood or quality of life will have been obtained from the case history. Taking measures of how the client feels their swallow impairment is impacting on their lives at the start of the assessment process will give a baseline measure that can be reviewed and monitored after treatment. This can be done through specific questions or rating scales. There are some formal quality of life measures available, such as the SWAL-QOL (McHorney et al., 2002) or the Dysphagia Handicap Index (Gustafsson and Tibbling, 1991).

Interpretation

As with communication assessments, it is important to be aware of the potential influencing factors of the context of the swallow assessment and to take these into account when interpreting the information. These include reported and perceived levels of fatigue and perceived comfort of the client. The environment of the swallow assessment may also be a contributing factor if it is different from the client's natural eating and drinking environment (e.g. hospital clinic versus home).

An assessment in a clinical setting, such as a radiology suite for VF or an outpatient clinic, reduces the environmental and anticipatory cueing of the pre-oral stage of the swallow, which can affect the rest of the swallow phases, especially with older people.

Symptoms of swallow impairment will have been observed and noted throughout assessment. Table 7.2 describes some differentiation between typical and more concerning symptoms. Some of these symptoms will only be visible through instrumental assessment, such as VF or FEES.

Table 7.2 Differentiation between typical and more concerning symptoms

Typical age-related symptoms of eating, drinking and swallowing impairment	Atypical/pathological symptoms associated with eating, drinking and swallowing
• Sense of smell slightly diminished • Taste changes with increasing preference for sweeter tastes • Some tooth loss or need for dentures • Slower chewing and avoidance of very hard or very chewy textures • Slow oral transfer • Some tongue weakness • Slower swallow initiation • Mild residue in the pharynx post swallow • Laryngeal penetration of bolus	• Sudden or profound loss of sense of smell or taste • Oral pain or infection • Anterior loss of food or fluid from the lips • Very slow oral transfer or holding food or fluid in the mouth • Food remaining in the lateral sulci between the teeth and cheeks • Nasal regurgitation of fluid or food • Significant tongue weakness • Significantly delayed swallow initiation • Widespread, significant residue of the bolus in the pharynx post swallow • Slow, ineffective closure of the airway • Coughing, voice change, breathlessness when eating or drinking signalling possible aspiration • Aspiration of food or fluids • Silent aspiration • Choking episodes

Whether the swallow impairment is age-related or have a more serious underlying cause will start to become evident during the assessment process and observation of symptoms. It may well be obvious that the swallow impairment is a dysphagia related to a disease if the client has had a recent stroke or has a diagnosis of dementia. Age-related swallow impairments are likely to display much milder symptoms than pathological dysphagia, and there are specific symptoms that would not be considered normal in age-related swallowing changes, as shown in Table 7.2. One of the clearest differences is that it is unlikely that persistent aspiration of food or fluids would occur with natural ageing, although penetration of food or fluids into the laryngeal vestibule is more likely with age.

Perhaps the most difficult to distinguish is the more severe age-related swallow changes versus dysphagia due to frailty. However, if there is severe age-related sarcopenia, this in itself is a high risk factor for loss of reserve and frailty, so this would also be a serious concern.

If the reason for swallow impairment is unclear, if there are atypical symptoms present or if there are additional swallow symptoms that do not fit with the current diagnosis, the clinician will need to look at the swallow symptoms and discern whether referral for further investigation is indicated. Table 7.3 details some of the more concerning patterns of swallow

Table 7.3   More concerning patterns of swallow impairment

Possible symptoms	Possible underlying cause	Further investigation / from whom to seek referral
Progressive dysphagia and overt symptoms impacting significantly on eating and drinking. **Red flags: dysarthria, limb weakness, nasal regurgitation of drink/food, tongue fasciculations and weight loss**	Progressive neurological disease	Neurology
Progressive dysphagia, may have pain on swallowing, patches of discolouration/ulceration in mouth or throat and lumps in mouth or neck. **Red flags: smoking, alcohol intake, associated voice changes and weight loss**	Head and neck cancers	ENT
Sudden onset of dysphagia symptoms. **Red flags: sudden communication difficulties, limb weakness and facial asymmetry**	Stroke TIA Brain haemorrhage	Urgent hospital care if symptoms have just developed. GP to urgently request referral for further investigations or neuroimaging, if these were not carried out when symptoms developed.
Forgetting to eat or drink, chewing excessively, holding food in the mouth, attempting to eat inedible items and having poor recognition of food/drink. **Red flags: associated cognition or memory impairment, and acute infection**	Delirium Dementia	GP/consultant in healthcare of older people Memory clinic Neurology
Poor oral intake, weight loss, reduced grip strength and reduced mobility, and slow walking speed. **Red flags: reduced ability to recover from infection and repeated infections**	Frailty	GP/consultant in healthcare of the older people
Food sticking and not going down, food more difficult to swallow than fluids, regurgitation of food or fluids and reflux. **Red flags: progressively deteriorating symptoms, alcohol intake and weight loss**	Oesophageal level impairments Oesophageal cancer Hiatus hernia Possible pharyngeal pouch	Gastroenterology for suspected oesophageal-level impairments ENT or imaging to investigate pharyngeal pouch

impairment, what these might mean and where the client may need referral to for further investigation. This is not an exhaustive list but contains the most common differential diagnoses that may occur in older people.

The additional challenge for clinicians working with older people is that there may well be pathological change occurring on the background of normal age-related change, so they are dealing with two aspects of swallow change.

Following the initial assessment, a hypothesis about the nature of the swallow impairment is usually formed, which in turn influences goal setting and intervention.

Goal setting and intervention

Content of client goals and method of intervention will arise from the interpretation of the assessment and any subsequent medical diagnoses that the client might receive following further investigation. The nature and consequences of the swallow impairment should be discussed frankly and sensitively with the client. Again, the word 'intervention' here is used to describe any swallow management strategies or rehabilitation plan.

The type of intervention needs to be a balance among the risk factors for aspiration pneumonia and choking (see Chapter 6), risk factors for increased sarcopenia and frailty, nature and severity (and prognosis) of the swallow impairment or disorder, and quality of life. We are aware that older people may have a baseline elevated vulnerability to aspiration pneumonia and increased risk of choking, and that the ageing process increases the risk for frailty. The type of intervention itself might also influence this. For instance, recommending avoiding or adapting some foods could lead to weight loss and increased sarcopenia if there is not sufficient dietetic support.

Quality of life is an important factor in the choice of intervention for swallow impairment. An older person with a progressive disorder who enjoys eating and drinking might decide not to have heavily modified food and drink, and accept the risk and consequences of aspiration pneumonia.

Diagram 7.1 is a summary of the factors that will influence the decision on goal setting and intervention through joint discussion with clients and sometimes their families or carers.

Following this is Table 7.4, which summarises common intervention techniques and considerations for older people. The reader is encouraged to study specific management techniques for

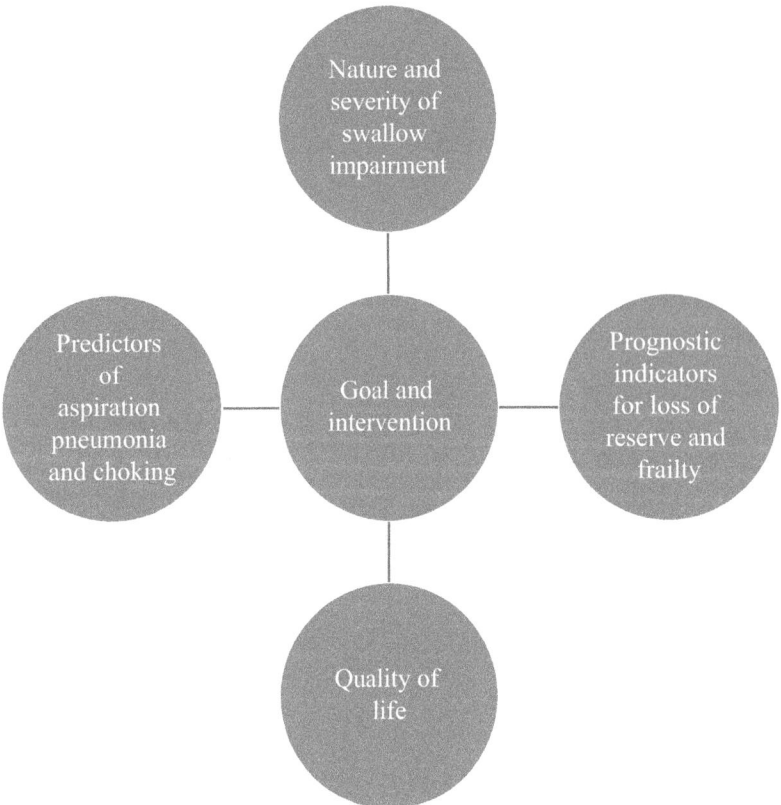

Diagram 7.1   *Factors that will influence the decision on goal setting and intervention*

Table 7.4   Common intervention techniques and considerations for older people

Method of intervention	Considerations for older adults
Education For example: Education of the cause and prognosis of the swallow impairment and the rationale behind the intervention choice, identifying symptoms that might indicate deterioration, lifestyle and risk factors	Education needs to be given to all people involved in the care of the older person, with their consent or documented best interest. Education on risk factors for aspiration pneumonia and choking, and lifestyle factors to slow the rate of sarcopenia are vital in optimising safety of the swallow and quality of life. There are information sheets available in the 'Resources' section covering various aspects of care for older people with swallow impairment.
Adaptations to the eating and drinking environment For example: Changing aspects of the environment to encourage safer eating and drinking Maximising cues in the pre-oral stage	The eating and drinking environment can be changeable for older people. There might be moves to a care home, a hospital admission or a move in with a family member. The ageing swallow is slower and weaker, and therefore, increasing cues in the pre-oral stage will boost the signals to the brain to help it prepare for the swallowing process. This is especially important if there has been a sudden change to the environment. An information sheet on optimising the environment for safer eating and drinking is in the 'Resources' section.

Method of intervention	Considerations for older adults
Feeding techniques For example: Pace of eating and drinking Type of utensil Finger foods to encourage self- feeding Hand-over-hand feeding is a method in which clients who are not able to feed themselves are encouraged to participate in the process with a carer's or family member's hand on theirs, guiding them as they use a utensil or cup	The speed of eating and drinking can cause some disruption as the swallow begins to age. An ageing slow swallow is not compatible with a fast pace of eating and drinking and can make it less safe. Older people need to be encouraged to feed themselves for as long as possible, as dependence on others for feeding is a key risk factor for developing aspiration pneumonia. Some carers might start to feed an older client so that they can finish the meal more quickly and take in more nutrition. However, if an older person is becoming slower to eat, it would be best to move to a little and often approach to eating and drinking so that the person can continue to self- feed smaller amounts to reduce the fatigue caused by feeding themselves a larger meal. Finger foods, such as fishfingers or cut-up sandwiches, can be a good prompt for an older person to self-feed and are especially effective for older people with a cognitive impairment so long as they can safely chew and swallow foods of that consistency. An advice leaflet on finger foods can be found in the 'Resources' section.
Modification of the food or fluid bolus For example: Changing the size, flavour or consistency of the bolus Thicker fluids might be recommended to increase sensory signals or to slow the passage of the fluid down to allow for optimal airway closure as the bolus passes through the pharynx Food may be modified to make it easier to chew and to reduce the risk of choking Any adaptations to the consistency of food or fluid need to relate to IDDSI (International Dysphagia Diet Standardisation Initiative); see Appendix 1	Sweeter flavours might produce a stronger sensory signal in older people than other flavours due to altering taste perception. There is evidence that carbonated drinks and sour flavours can also provide increased sensory stimulation to improve swallow function (Loret, 2015). Modifying the consistency of food and drinks is relatively common practice for SLTs in managing swallow impairment, although requires a benefits-versus-risk assessment for each individual. It is important to be aware of the potential impact this could have on nutrition and hydration as well as quality of life. The risk of aspiration pneumonia and choking needs to be balanced with nutrition and hydration factors as well as the client's quality of life. This often depends on the client's medical diagnosis and prognosis. Flavoured thickened drinks can improve sensory awareness as well as slowing the bolus down to allow for slower movements of the swallow structure. Modified food is easier to chew, which helps if the chewing is slower and can also reduce risk of choking. Consideration needs to be given to how the modified meals or thickened drinks will be prepared at home if clients are unable to do this for themselves. There is an information sheet on how to fortify food to maximise calorie intake in the 'Resources' section of this chapter. Visual appearance of modified meals needs to be considered as well as taste. Optimising the visual appearance will encourage increased oral intake and enhance pre-oral cues.

(Continued)

Table 7.4 (Continued)

Method of intervention	Considerations for older adults
Specific postures, strategies and exercises There are a range of specific head postures, swallow strategies and exercises that are recommended to manage particular swallow concerns. These are advised by the SLT following detailed assessment of the individual and often recommended following an instrumental assessment where the effects of these can be visualised. These interventions might be compensatory in the case of some head postures, which aim to optimise the safe passage of the bolus, or rehabilitative, such as tongue strengthening exercises or expiratory muscle strength training.	There is variable evidence on the use of exercises for swallow rehabilitation (Langmore and Pisegna, 2015), and the effects of the exercises might be different for older people. Any contraindications to swallow exercises and strategies need to be considered. Some techniques, such as the breath-hold-swallow (super or supraglottic swallow) is contraindicated in clients with cardiac issues or hypertension. Some compensatory head postures might be difficult for older people with arthritis or any neck complaints. There is evidence for tongue strengthening exercises for healthy older people with age-related sarcopenia (Yano et al., 2020; Robbins et al., 2005) and with frailty (Lopez et al., 2018). There are devices to measure tongue strength and provide training exercises. Not all services have access to these. There is an example sheet of basic tongue resistance exercises in the 'Resources' section. There is some evidence that expiratory muscle strength training with older people has some effect on strength of the swallow muscles and can lead to enhanced cough function (Kim et al., 2009; Ito et al., 2017). There could well be fatigue effects for older people who are frail or who have poor nutritional intake, and this needs to be taken account when deciding on an exercise regime. Older people with cognitive impairment may have more difficulty learning or recalling strategies and exercises. Written information and prompting can help.

dysphagia related to disease but to keep in mind these considerations as they are dealing with an ageing swallow alongside a disease-induced dysphagia. There are two case studies at the end of the chapter that demonstrate this type of goal setting and intervention planning.

Non-oral feeding in older adults

In the event of a person's swallow becoming so unsafe that food, drink and medications all carry a high risk of aspiration and choking and/or in the circumstance of not being able to meet nutritional or hydration needs orally, methods of non-oral feeding are a consideration. The most common means of non-oral feeding is via a tube, either a temporary tube, such as a nasogastric (NG) tube or a more permanent percutaneous endoscopic gastrostomy (PEG), or radiologically inserted gastrostomy (RIG).

The decision of whether a person is fed via a tube should not be made based on age but rather on the basis of medical diagnosis and prognosis, expectations of swallow recovery, and quality of life and fitness for the procedure.

A multidisciplinary discussion is required involving the client on the risk versus benefits of oral feeding with risk of aspiration pneumonia and choking versus the risks and benefits of non-oral feeding.

Some older people take the view that they will accept the risks of aspiration pneumonia if they can continue to eat and drink food they enjoy. Other older people might be distressed by their aspiration symptoms and might wish to explore the option of tube feeding to provide their nutritional requirements alongside smaller, safer quantities of food intake orally. Longer-term feeding tubes, such as a PEG or a RIG, require someone to be able to administer the feeds and maintain the tube, so this also needs to be considered.

Outcomes

As in the case of communication intervention, measuring outcomes for treatment of swallow impairment will vary. Many services will choose their outcome measures as one which measures client outcomes but also enables them to collect data for the requirements of the wider organisation.

Revisiting the client's initial goals and how these have been met can be an effective, individual-focused outcome measure. For example, have the symptoms of swallow impairment reduced? Are the risk factors for aspiration pneumonia reduced? If the client has a terminal, progressive disease, the outcomes might focus more on comfort and reduction of distressing symptoms. Any formal questionnaires can be repeated and results compared.

Follow-up

Do we routinely follow up older clients with a phone call or face-to-face appointment, or discharge them from the service and await re-referral following an episode of care? One argument for routine follow-up of these clients is that any symptoms of age-related swallow impairment may be masking the early signs of disease-related dysphagia. The older person's swallow is also more vulnerable to loss of reserve and frailty than the swallow of younger counterparts and so requires more monitoring.

The service availability might not be compatible with routine check-up appointments. A triage system could be set up, looking at the prognostic indicators for ongoing risk of dysphagia with the highest scorers receiving a formal follow-up. If not receiving a formal follow-up appointment, it is a necessity that the client and/or their family receive education on signs and symptoms to watch out for, and know how to action a referral back into the service as required.

Case examples

Case example 1

Jakub is a 75-year-old man admitted to the hospital with a urinary tract infection (UTI) and confusion. He was referred to speech and language therapy for a swallow assessment after a choking episode on meat. Nursing staff on the ward had also noticed him occasionally coughing when drinking.

Background: Jakub has no history of swallowing difficulty and no medical diagnoses apart from a small stroke 20 years ago, which he recovered well from. He takes medication for hypertension. He lives independently and cooks his own meals. He and his daughter report that he has always tended to eat and drink very quickly, but the coughing episodes are new. He had started to lose some weight in the months prior to hospital admission. Jakub is responding to treatment for his UTI, and he has become less confused. His chest has remained clear throughout admission, and he is now walking around the ward.

Assessment:

   Bedside swallow assessment: Jakub was sitting upright in the chair beside his bed, alert and talking.

   Cranial nerve assessment: There were no observed cranial nerve deficiencies apart from slight left-sided facial weakness from previous stroke. Oral check indicated dry, coated tongue and loose dentures.

   Oral trials of water (200mls): Jakub drank this quickly with consecutive swallows. Subjectively, laryngeal movement felt slow. There was a throat clear and cough at the end of the drink.

   Mealtime observation (jacket potato with cheese and beans): Jakub was eating quickly and putting large amounts in his mouth before chewing. Some difficulty chewing the skin of the potato and taking this out of his mouth.

Interpretation: Likely age-related sarcopenia and loss of reserve due to current infection, meaning that there is reduced airway protection on swallowing and the swallow is less able to respond to the speed of eating and drinking. Loose dentures are affecting the oral phase of the swallow. There may be some residual weakness from previous stroke.

> *Risk factors for aspiration/choking*: Speed of eating and drinking, loose dentures.
>
> *Risk factors for aspiration pneumonia:* Poor oral hygiene.
>
> *Risk factors for loss of reserve / frailty*: Swallow appears to be vulnerable to loss of reserve. There was some weight loss prior to hospital admission, which could impact on nutritional status.
>
> *Quality of life*: Loose dentures may be affecting ability to chew foods and the need to avoid certain foods.

Goal setting: Discussed with Jakub and his daughter.

- To refer to the medical team for investigation into current weight loss to check for any underlying issues and to the dietitian for weight management.
- To reduce the risk of choking.
- To reduce the episodes of coughing when drinking (reducing aspiration risk).
- To educate about good mouthcare to reduce the risk of aspiration pneumonia.

Intervention: Jakub and his daughter were encouraged to visit his dentist for assessment and advice regarding dentures, and to use a denture fixing gel during mealtimes in the meantime. He was advised to avoid very chewy or hard foods and tough fruit or vegetable skins.

Strategies were given to help pace eating and drinking, including cutting food up prior to the meal and encouraging him to take one piece at a time to chew and swallow before taking the next. He was also encouraged to take one sip at a time when drinking rather than continuous drinking. He was given written prompts for these strategies, which he kept on his table.

Education and leaflets were given on mouthcare, and the association between poor oral hygiene and aspiration pneumonia was discussed. They were given the 'High-risk foods' leaflet as a reminder of which foods carry a high choking risk and the 'Getting more out of your food drink' leaflet for advice on getting more calories from food pending the dietitian appointment (see the 'Resources' section for these leaflets).

Outcome: Jakub took time to adopt the strategies of eating and drinking more slowly, but encouraging him to cut his food up helped to remind him as well as reminding him to read the written advice. Drinking more slowly reduced the episodes of coughing when drinking. The denture fixing gel helped his dentures to fit better at mealtimes pending his dentist appointment. He avoided or took extra care with high-risk foods. There have been no further choking episodes and no chest infections.

His tongue was less coated and dry, and he was encouraged to continue good mouthcare on his return home.

Review: As Jakub was able to eat and drink with no significant concerns, he was not referred to the Community SLT. However, he was advised that his swallow might be vulnerable, and his risk of aspiration and/or choking may increase if he becomes unwell in the future. It also cannot be ruled out that his swallow might change over time or that these symptoms may have been the start of a progressive dysphagia. Jakub and his daughter were educated on symptoms of dysphagia and advised to seek referral to SLT if any of these are noted in future. If his swallow symptoms return or get worse, or if he starts to get chest infections, a referral for a more detailed objective swallow assessment, such as a videofluoroscopy, may be indicated.

Case example 2

Joan is 91 years old and has recently moved to a care home near her family. The staff at the home have referred her to SLT for a swallow assessment with concern that she is reluctant to eat and drink, and she is holding food in her mouth.

Background: Joan lived in alone in her own home for 20 years following the death of her husband. She was diagnosed with dementia three years ago. At home, she would heat up basic meals and eat them sitting in her armchair with a tray. She can engage well in conversation if she is able to choose and lead the topic but has difficulty with new topics. She made the decision alongside her family to move into a care home with the knowledge that her dementia symptoms are increasingly affecting her ability to manage at home.

Her other medical diagnosis is osteoarthritis. She has not had any recent chest infections. She has lost weight since moving to the care home. Staff report that she often holds food in her mouth, and they have started to try and feed her as she is reluctant to feed herself.

Assessment: Assessment was informal and included cranial nerve assessment and mealtime observation at the care home.

Joan was able to copy some of the movements for the cranial nerve assessment. Tongue movement was slightly slow, but there were no obvious cranial nerve deficiencies. Oral hygiene was good. Joan has her own teeth, which are in reasonable condition.

Mealtime observation: Joan is eating a meal in the dining room with several other residents around the table. Joan appeared distracted by the noises and people around her. She had sandwiches on her plate, and she appeared to forget these were there. The staff cut the sandwiches into small squares and fed them to her. Joan chewed the sandwich for a little while and then held it in her mouth and needed prompts to keep chewing and swallowing. She fed herself a few spoons of yoghurt for dessert.

Interpretation: It appears likely that Joan's change in routine and eating environment has influenced the pre-oral phase of her swallowing. She is not receiving the same cues to prompt her to start eating and drinking. Limitations in the pre-oral stage might be leading to holding food in the mouth in the oral stage.

> *Risk factors for aspiration/choking*: Holding food in the mouth. Residue in the mouth after meals could be a risk factor for aspiration/choking. Reduced sensory and motor cues in the pre-oral stage may affect the pharyngeal phase of swallow. Distracted by other people in the dining room.
>
> *Risk factors for aspiration pneumonia:* Staff are feeding Joan, so she is dependent for feeding.
>
> *Risk factors for loss of reserve and frailty:* Losing weight. Reduced mobility.
>
> *Quality of life:* Quality of life may have been affected by change of eating and drinking environment. Independence has been reduced by needing to be fed by staff members.

Goals: Overall aims are to increase Joan's oral intake and optimise the safety of her swallowing.

- To help Joan become more familiar with the eating and drinking environment.
- To increase sensory cues for eating and drinking in the pre-oral stage of swallowing.
- To establish independent or near-independent feeding.
- To educate staff on the risk factors for aspiration pneumonia.

Intervention: A series of interventions were put in place through discussion with Joan and her family. She was initially put on a smaller table in a quieter area with just a few other residents to reduce distractions and then moved to a quieter area of the main dining hall when she was used to having people around her.

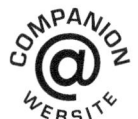

Sensory cues were increased by putting cutlery in her hands to lay out at the table, her daughter brought in some of her familiar plates and cups, and she was also given some coloured plates to help with visual recognition of food. Staff played familiar music at mealtimes to signal the time of day.

Different flavours of food were tried, and Joan appeared to respond better to stronger flavours. She liked to have tomato sauce with meals and preferred sweet fillings to sandwiches, such as jam. The increased sensory signal of these flavours seemed to prompt her to chew and not hold food in her mouth.

Staff were taught hand-over-hand feeding with their hand over Joan's on the fork or spoon to help her to engage with the motor patterns for feeding to strengthen the sequencing of the swallow phases and reduce the risk of aspiration pneumonia. As Joan became more focused during mealtimes, she started to feed herself more and would regularly feed herself with finger foods, such as fishfingers and chips.

Staff were educated on the symptoms of dysphagia and the risk factors for aspiration pneumonia. They continued to promote good oral hygiene and reduce dependency for feeding.

Outcome: Joan's oral intake increased, and she managed to eat nearly all her meals at each mealtime. She appeared more comfortable and less distracted in the new eating environment. Her swallow appeared safer as she was not holding food in her mouth so often, and her risk factors for aspiration pneumonia were reduced.

In line with Joan's dementia diagnosis, it is likely that her swallowing ability will deteriorate in the coming months and years. Staff at the care home are aware of symptoms to watch out for and how to re-refer to SLT if there are future concerns.

Resources

- Diary of eating, drinking and swallowing symptoms
- Eating, drinking, and swallowing case history proforma
- General eating and drinking advice for older people
- Tips for a good mouthcare regime
- Getting more out of your food and drink
- Optimising the environment for safer eating and drinking: Information for carers
- Finger foods
- High-risk foods
- Tongue resistance exercises

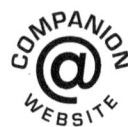

Diary of eating, drinking and swallowing symptoms

- Please document the food or drink that you have at each mealtime or snack time across one week (see Table 7.5).
- Circle any foods or drink that you have any difficulty with.
- Describe the difficulty you are experiencing. Symptoms may include but are not limited to coughing or throat clearing, choking feeling, feeling breathless, feeling of food or fluid being stuck, difficulty chewing, food or liquid coming back out of the mouth or down the nose, difficulty achieving a swallow and food staying in your mouth after swallowing.
- Note any details that might be relevant (e.g. mood, tiredness levels, eating environment, and eating alone or with other people).
- **Please bring this completed form to your appointment on this date:**

Table 7.5 Diary of eating, drinking and swallowing symptoms

	Breakfast	Lunch	Dinner	Drinks	Snacks	Symptoms	Other details
Sat							
Sun							
Mon							
Tues							
Weds							
Thurs							
Fri							

Eating, drinking and swallowing case history proforma

Table 7.6 Eating, drinking and swallowing case history proforma

Name DOB NHS no
Reason for referral
Past medical history

(Continued)

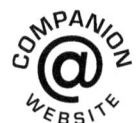

Table 7.6 (Continued)

Medication / side effects
Smoking status
Alcohol intake
Recent medical investigations
Visual/hearing impairment
Client account of swallow impairment
Nature of onset of impairment (e.g. sudden, occasional or chronic, and speed of deterioration)
Dental/oral hygiene (e.g. denture wearer, health of own teeth and oral hygiene routine)
Recent or recurring chest infections
Ability to eat balanced diet / weight management
Food shopping and meal preparation
Impact of swallow impairment on quality of life
Strategies client is already using
Expectations of appointment / client goals around swallowing

General eating and drinking advice for older people

The process of eating, drinking and swallowing changes naturally as we get older. Our appetites can change, and there are small changes to our smell and taste. If there is reduced overall strength and fitness, the muscles of chewing and swallowing can become weak. This

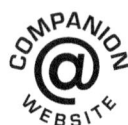

can increase the risk of choking and chest infections from food or drink going down the wrong way into the airway.

Here are some general tips for safer eating and drinking in older age:

- Focus and take time to chew and swallow carefully when eating.
- Try not to put too much food in your mouth at once and cut large pieces of food (e.g. meat) into smaller pieces before eating.
- Avoid very hard or very chewy foods, especially if you have dentures or poor dentition.
- Try to eat a balanced diet, although follow any individual diet plans if you have been given one by a healthcare professional.
- Try to keep up with physical fitness, as this can reduce the rate of muscle loss.
- Keep a note of and avoid any foods you find difficult to chew or swallow.
- Sip water regularly, avoid very dry foods or moisten foods with sauces if your mouth is feeling dry. Your doctor or pharmacist may be able to advise you on products to moisten your mouth depending on the reason for the dry mouth.

If you have any concerns regarding your eating and drinking (e.g. if you are having to avoid more and more foods), if the symptoms are getting worse, or if you are coughing or choking when eating or drinking, please contact your doctor.

Tips for a good mouthcare regime

Poor oral hygiene and tooth decay can cause discomfort and pain, and are linked with several serious conditions, such as an increased risk of pneumonia, heart disease and stroke.

Taking time to establish a thorough oral care routine can help to prevent tooth loss and pain as well as reduce the risk of more serious illness.

Tips for a good oral care routine include the following:

- Brush your teeth twice a day using a fluoride toothpaste.
- Use a soft- to medium-headed toothbrush.
- Brush all surfaces of your teeth and where the teeth meet your gums.
- Brush your tongue as well as brushing your teeth.
- Floss between your teeth daily.
- Spit out the toothpaste rather than rinsing your mouth out after brushing.
- Reduce sugar intake.

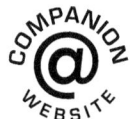

- Attend regular dental check-ups.
- Look out for any abnormalities in your mouth, such as lumps, any patches of discolouration or ulcers that do not heal. Contact your doctor if you notice these symptoms or any other unusual symptoms.

References

Take Care of Your Teeth and Gums. www.nhs.uk
Mouthcare Matters Resources. www.mouthcarematters.hee.nhs.uk/links-resources

Getting more out of your food and drink

If you have a poor appetite or are too tired or unwell to cook full meals, you can help maintain or gain weight by naturally fortifying your food with high-calorie items without the pressure to eat more. Having small, regular high-calorie meals or snacks throughout the day might be easier than having three large meals a day.

Foods that can be used to naturally fortify your meals, snacks or drinks are listed subsequently. This advice is aimed at people who are struggling to maintain or gain weight. It is essential that any unintentional weight loss is investigated by a doctor who may also refer you to a dietitian. If you have been asked to stick to a particular diet or to have a certain consistency of food because of a swallowing difficulty, please check with the relevant health professional before following the advice in this leaflet.

Naturally fortifying foods:

Whole or full-fat milk

Full-fat spread or butter

Cream (especially double cream)

Full-fat cheese

Full-fat mayonnaise

Sugar

Jam

Honey

Syrup

Chocolate spread

Dried fruit

Condensed milk

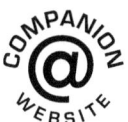

Optimising the environment for safer eating and drinking: Information for carers

The eating and drinking environment can impact directly on the eating and drinking process, and the ability to swallow safely. The body takes clues from the environment via our senses to prepare for eating and drinking. For example, the smell of cooking increases saliva production, which in turn helps with efficient chewing.

With advancing age, our bodies need more of these environmental cues. This is especially the case with people who have dementia or who have suddenly changed their eating and drinking environment due to a move to a care home or a hospital admission.

Here are some strategies that can help optimise the eating and drinking environment to promote a better appetite and safer swallowing:

- Try to keep routines around times of meals and places where the meal takes place.
- Set out utensils for eating and drinking in advance of the meal.
- Signal mealtimes by playing familiar music in the background so this music is associated with eating and drinking. Listening to familiar music whilst eating can help increase food intake (Thomas and Smith, 2009).
- Use coloured plates to improve the visual perception of the food in contrast to the plate (Dunne et al., 2004).
- Encourage looking at and smelling the meal before starting to eat.
- Consider that familiar food associated with comforting memories might help stimulate appetite.
- Try hand-over-hand feeding with your hand over theirs on the utensil or cup to encourage engagement in the process if the person needs assistance with eating and drinking.
- Eat with other people around a table to help stimulate appetite so long as there are not too many distractions.
- Ask if you can take items, such as a familiar cup or plate or placemat as visual reminders of mealtimes, if there is a change of environment, such as a hospital admission.

If you notice any symptoms of swallowing difficulty, such as coughing when eating or drinking, choking episodes, or unintentional weight loss, please contact the doctor for further investigation.

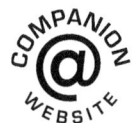

References

Dunne, TE, Neagarder, SA et al. (2004) Visual contrast enhances food and liquid intake in advanced Alzheimer's disease. *Clinical Nutrition*. 4: 533–538, August 23.

Thomas, D and Smith, M (2009) The effect of music on calorie consumption among nursing home residents with dementia of the Alzheimer's type. *Activities, Adaptation and Aging*. 33 (1): 1–16.

Finger foods

Finger foods are food items that can be picked up and eaten without much mess. If people are struggling with their appetite, finger foods can help them eat little and often rather than be overwhelmed by a full plate of food at mealtimes. Finger foods can also help to maintain independent eating and drinking for people who have difficulty using utensils.

Here is a list of examples of finger foods. If a certain diet or special consistency of food has been recommended by a healthcare professional (dietitian or speech and language therapist, for example), please check with the healthcare professional which of these foods would be suitable in these cases, as some of these foods could cause harm.

Fishfingers

Sandwiches cut into small pieces

Naan bread / chapatti / pitta bread / toast cut into strips

Small pizza slices

Sausage roll

Scotch egg

Samosa

Onion bhaji

Chips

Hard-boiled egg

Crisps

Nuts

Pieces of fruit

Dried fruit

Vegetable sticks

Crackers

High-risk foods

High-risk foods are foods that are typically difficult to chew and swallow. These carry a higher risk of choking or getting stuck in the throat. They can be particularly difficult if you

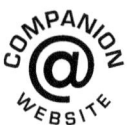

do not have many teeth or if you have ill-fitting dentures. These foods also carry a risk for people with swallowing disorders.

Some of these foods can be adapted to make them safer to swallow. For example, dry crumble can be mixed with custard. Please follow any specific swallowing or dietary advice that has been recommended to you by health professionals.

Some examples of high-risk foods are listed subsequently. Please add to the list any other foods that are difficult for you to chew and swallow. If you notice that your swallowing symptoms are getting worse (e.g. if the list of foods is getting longer, if you are coughing when eating or drinking, or if you notice any unintentional weight loss), please contact your doctor.

- Crumbly, dry textures (e.g. crumble, crackers, rice, dry biscuits and flaky pastry)
- Chewy foods (e.g. chewy meat, chewy sweets, dried fruit and bread crusts)
- Mixed liquid and solid (e.g. soup with food pieces or croutons, cereal and milk, and oranges)
- Large lumps of food (e.g. meat in large pieces and chewy bread crusts)
- Hard foods (e.g. boiled sweets, nuts and some crisps)
- Foods with skins (e.g. grapes, sausages and cucumber)
- Fibrous, stringy foods (e.g. lettuce, runner beans and corn on the cob)

Tongue resistance exercises

Tongue strength starts to weaken in older age. This happens naturally and can occur to varying degrees depending on lifestyle factors, such as nutritional intake and general fitness. A weaker tongue can lead to problems with swallowing, such as the ability to move the food to the back of the mouth ready for swallowing or the strength to swallow food down into the food pipe.

Here are some exercises to help improve tongue strength. Your clinician will advise you on which of these are relevant for you.

Try to practise regularly throughout the day.

Repeat each exercise five times.

- Push the tip of your tongue against a flat object, such as a tongue depressor or the long end of a spoon, directly in front of your mouth. Push it away with your tongue.

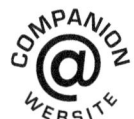

- Stick out your tongue and push the tip of your tongue upwards against the flat object just above your mouth.
- Stick out your tongue and put the flat object to one side of your tongue. Press against it with the side of your tongue. Repeat on the other side.

References

DePippo, KL, Holas, MA and Reding MJ (1992) Validation of the 3oz water test for aspiration following stroke. *Archives of Neurology*. 49: 1259-1261.

Gustafsson, B and Tibbling, L (1991) Dysphagia, an unrecognised handicap. *Dysphagia*. 6: 193-199.

Ito, N et al. (2017) The effect of expiratory muscle strength training on the swallow function of the elderly. *Innovation in Aging: The Gerontological Society of America*. 1 (Supp 1): 230-231.

Kim, J, Davenport, P and Sapienza, C (2009) Effect of expiratory muscle strength training on elderly cough function. *Archives of Gerontology and Geriatrics*. 48 (3): 361-366.

Langmore, SE and Pisegna, JM (2015) Efficacy of exercises to rehabilitate dysphagia: A critique of the literature. *International Journal of Speech and Language Pathology*. 17 (3): 222-229.

Langmore, SE et al. (1998) Predictors of aspiration pneumonia: How important is dysphagia? *Dysphagia*. 13: 69-81.

Lopez, P et al. (2018) Benefits of resistance training in physically frail elderly. *Aging Clinical and Experimental Research*. 8: 889-899, August 30.

Loret, C (2015) Using sensory properties of food to trigger swallowing: A review. *Clinical Reviews in Food Science and Nutrition*. 255 (1): 140-145.

McHorney, C et al. (2002) SWAL-QOL and SWAL-CARE outcome tools for oro-pharyngeal dysphagia in adults III: Documentation of reliability and validity. *Dysphagia*. 17: 97-114.

Robbins, J et al. (2005) The effects of lingual exercise on swallowing in older adults. *Journal of the American Geriatric Society*. 53 (9): 1483-1489.

Yano, J et al. (2020) Effects of tongue strengthening self exercises in healthy older adults: A non-randomised control trial. *Dysphagia*. 36 (5), November 19.

DECISION MAKING IN LATER LIFE

DOI: 10.4324/9781003058090-9

Introduction

Older age can bring forth significant lifestyle changes that require serious thought and decision making.

Such considerations in older age can include the following:

- **Accommodation:** whether to downsize, move closer to family, move closer to amenities and/or medical facilities, make adaptations to current accommodation, and move into a care or nursing institution.
- **Financial:** considering when to retire, budgeting of pension, managing wills and choosing a person to take responsibility over financial decisions in the event of not being able to.
- **Health:** risk versus benefits of medications, advanced decision making, appointment of someone to take responsibility for health decisions in the event of not being able to, and statement of wishes around medical care and intervention, including those around hospital admissions and preferred place of death.

Some people prefer to plan for these changes in advance. For example, a person might downsize to a smaller house to reduce the need to have to do this in the case of physical decline in older age or plan to move to a new house to be closer to family in the event of needing more support in later years. Other people prefer to take life as it comes and will decide to downsize if physical decline becomes an issue.

Advanced planning can be difficult, as it relies on the older person having to envisage a time when they may be more dependent on people for care and less able to do activities they are currently able to do. This can bring a sense of fear and trepidation. However, there are benefits to planning for the future. These include moving to a new house whilst being physically and cognitively able, and therefore, being able to create new social networks, having control over decision making and having the opportunity to state future wishes.

Influencing factors might be the experience of witnessing the needs of a family member or friend in older age, personality type or family involvement.

Early planning is often precipitated by the diagnosis of a terminal or chronic illness. The trajectory of these illnesses, such as terminal cancer or motor neurone disease, is relatively clearly defined, and therefore, decisions, such as treatment plans or end of life care, can be made in advance with the support of a healthcare professional.

The pattern of decline in natural ageing is less clear but, with or without a health diagnosis, will eventually lead to death and arguably requires a similar type of planning that is offered to people who are diagnosed with a terminal illness. The process of discussing and documenting whether an older person would like to be resuscitated in the event of a cardiac arrest is common and well documented. Other types of advanced care planning for older people are also gaining ground. However, the best time to introduce these conversations is a challenge, especially if the person does not have a health diagnosis. This is discussed in more detail in the next section.

This topic is especially relevant to clinicians working with older people. Although healthcare professionals support care planning and decision making with clients of all ages and diagnoses, there is increased prevalence of significant health and lifestyle change in older age and the increased risk of losing cognitive ability to make complex choices through illness, such as dementia.

The decision making process is rarely black and white, even with seemingly straightforward choices. Often, either choice can lead to some negative consequences, and there are choices within choices and emotional responses to consider. Examples include an older person choosing to stay at home but risking a serious fall, or an older person moving closer to family for care needs but leaving behind old friendships and a familiar environment. Emotions can overtake logic at times. Supporting an older person to make an informed decision requires time, careful and sensitive thought, and planning on behalf of clinicians.

This chapter will discuss topics around decision making in later life, including topics such as advanced care planning and mental capacity. There are links to communication and swallowing impairment with sections on how communication impairment affects the ability to make formal decisions and decisions that might need to be made by people with swallow impairment. There are case studies throughout the chapter to illustrate how this relates to clinical practice when working with older people with communication or swallow impairments.

Advanced care planning

In health terms, advanced care planning or advanced decision making is a method of putting plans in place according to people's preferences and wishes to cover potential health scenarios. As mentioned previously, it is mostly associated with palliative care or the diagnosis of a terminal illness when the healthcare team discuss with the client and family about putting these plans in place. It is a way of ensuring a person's wishes and preferences are documented if they become too unwell, lose consciousness or lose the mental capacity to make these decisions.

Advanced care planning is good practice in terms of planning for individualised care. As mentioned earlier, the timing of when is best to start these conversations with older people is not clear. This is especially in the case of very old people who are naturally moving towards death but could still have some control and engagement in planning for these last few years. Older people may have informally discussed some of their wishes with family members, but unless they have a specific health diagnosis, they are usually unlikely to come in to contact with healthcare professionals to document these more formally. It is often a hospital admission that starts to prompt these decisions, which by then may be too late in terms of the older person being able to engage with the decision making and what choices they may have.

Decision making for advanced care planning needs to be done on an informed basis where the individual is informed about the nature of the choices presented and the possible consequences of what each choice might lead to. Some people may have not thought about aspects of the decisions they are being asked to make and so might need some time to think. Poppe et al. (2013) looked at advanced care planning for people with early dementia and found that only one-third of patients interviewed had thought about any aspects of their future before these care planning discussions.

These discussions are ideally done with a healthcare professional and one who the client is familiar with. Poppe et al. (2013) found that staff felt that they were able to better facilitate advanced care planning decisions when they had a good relationship with the client and their family.

Types of considerations for advanced care planning with older people include the following:

- Medical intervention; for example, intravenous fluids, antibiotics and feeding tubes
- Pain management
- Admission to hospital
- Moving into a care or nursing home
- End of life care and preferred place of death

But advanced wishes can also contain preferences on other things that are important to people, such as food and drink likes and dislikes, music tastes, clothing tastes, and sensory needs (Age UK, 2021).

Cultural and spiritual needs and preferences also need to be accounted for. There may be certain beliefs about medical intervention in some circumstances. Some people would like to be visited by a chaplain and receive prayer. There may be certain rituals or traditions that people would like documented as being important to them.

The documentation of these wishes are not legally binding and need to be reviewed regularly. It may be that the individual feels one way when the advanced care planning is first discussed but may change these views as their illness progresses or with increasing age.

There are legal documents to support advanced care planning, and these have different titles depending on the country. Jurisdiction around these documents also varies, so these will not be discussed in detail. Currently in the UK, there is the option of creating a legal living will or an advanced directive to refuse treatment. This can include treatment that is life sustaining, with the knowledge that refusal of it could lead to death (NHS Advanced decisions (living will) 2020). They need to be written and signed by the person and a witness.

Examples of treatment refusal could include interventions, such as mechanical ventilation or the use of feeding tubes. They need to be specific and to be clear about which situations the refusal for treatment might cover. A person who enjoys eating and drinking might want to refuse a feeding tube in the event of a chronic unsafe swallow in older age, but they may accept one in the short term if they are involved in a serious car accident and unable to have food and drink orally for a temporary period.

Again, it is important to remember that even strongly held personal views can change, and these documents need to be discussed with the individual on a regular basis to check they still feel the same way.

In planning for older age, some people will designate a trusted family member or friend to be able to make decisions for them in the event of them being unable to make decisions due to reduced cognitive ability or loss of consciousness. This can be documented formally and legally in a process to make that trusted person a power of attorney. A power of attorney can be for financial or health decisions, or both, and may be temporary or long-lasting. A person needs to have sufficient mental capacity to be able to appoint a power of attorney.

Mental capacity

The risk of leaving advanced care decisions until later in age or until a crisis prompts a hospital admission is that a person might lose the mental capacity to make such decisions and, therefore, might not be able to have as much control over the process. Jethwa et al. (2015) report that advanced care planning becomes more of a challenge when individuals do not have the cognition to be able to make their own decisions.

Poppe et al. (2013) state that although advanced care planning should be discussed before people lose capacity to make decisions, it is not yet established routine practice with people who have dementia.

Assessment of mental capacity and the jurisdiction surrounding these assessments will again vary from country to country and is likely to change over time so will be discussed here in broad terms. The mental capacity of an individual to make a decision might be called into question if the person has a cognitive and/or severe communication impairment. This could arise from conditions, such as dementia or delirium, a stroke or head injury, or a severe learning disability. The cognitive impairment may be temporary or permanent. A state of unconsciousness would also render a person unable to make important decisions.

The UK Mental Capacity Act (2005) states that to demonstrate the cognitive ability to make a decision, the person needs to be able to do the following:

- Understand the information specific to the decision in question.
- Be able to retain this information.
- Carefully consider or use the information related to the decision in their decision making process.

(Mental Capacity Act, www.nhs.uk)

The person who is making the decision needs to have support to be able to understand and retain the relevant information, and be facilitated to be able to communicate their process of making the choice, including the potential consequences. This is explained further in the next section of the chapter on supporting people with communication impairment to make decisions.

It is important to note that mental capacity can also fluctuate in that a person can demonstrate the mental capacity to make a particular decision on one day but maybe not the next. This might be the case, for example, with an older person experiencing confusion or delirium because of an infection or fluctuating cognitive ability in the early stages of dementia. Mental capacity for decision making rests on particular decisions, so someone might demonstrate the mental capacity to wear a T-shirt outside in cold weather and weigh up the pros and cons of this but might not be able to demonstrate the mental capacity to make complex financial decisions.

The UK Mental Capacity Act (2005, www. legislation.gov.uk) allows for unwise decisions, which are decisions that a person has demonstrated the mental capacity to choose but are considered unwise. For example, an older person being able to understand, retain the information and weigh up the risks of staying at home with a treatable illness but deciding not to be admitted to hospital for intravenous antibiotics.

If a person does not demonstrate the mental capacity to make a particular decision and does not have an appointed power of attorney that covers that specific decision area (health or financial), a best-interest decision can be made, weighing up what is least distressing for the person, any previously declared or currently declared preferences and the overall context of the decision, such as medical prognosis. If the person's liberty, independence or freedom has been restricted as a result of decisions, there are legal frameworks that need to be put in place to ensure that this restriction is appropriate, proportionate and in the best interests of that individual and their circumstances. As a disclaimer, broad terms and examples have been used here, although with reference to the current UK Mental Capacity Act (2005). There are legal processes that are required for formal advanced decision making or refusal of treatment and for the carrying out and interpretation of mental capacity assessments. Readers need to be aware of the most recent legislation and adhere to this in their area of work.

Impact of communication impairment on decision making

The presence of a communication impairment adds a complexity to decision making In terms of the person being able to demonstrate understanding of the information involved and having the ability to clearly express the process of the decision making using the information related to the decision. This can be particularly difficult if the language related to the decision is complex or abstract.

Zuscak et al. (2015) report that decision making regarding legal decisions often require understanding of more complex spoken and written information than would be required for everyday matters. They make the important case that whilst people with communication disorders are likely to be compromised in their ability to understand and make important decisions, this is their human right, and they need as much support as possible to facilitate the process.

The onset of communication disorders is more likely to be in older age, with the increased prevalence of stroke, dementia and other neurological disorders. Therefore, there is some benefit to people being able to express their wishes and preferences or formally document them in a legal document earlier in life if they have strong feelings about what they would wish for in later life scenarios.

Mental capacity for specific decisions is decided on the basis of cognitive ability. Although it is understood that communication impairment can occur independently of a cognitive impairment, it can nevertheless be difficult to assess pure cognitive ability without accessing communication channels. Cognitive assessments tend to involve language-based questions, and verbal expression is a way of demonstrating the level of underlying cognitive processes.

It is important to have a good understanding of both a person's overall language ability and cognitive ability before broaching conversations about decision making. Ideally this would be done in a joint assessment with a speech and language therapist (SLT) to assess speech, language and communication, and an occupational therapist (OT) to assess cognition. There may be other professionals involved, such as a neuropsychologist, who can also assess cognition. Cognition may need to be assessed in more creative ways due to the language barrier. One example of this could be looking at how a person problem solves in functional activities, which do not require language. Talking to family members or other professionals involved with the care of the person can help understand how choices are communicated on a day-to-day basis. Age-related communication change, such as slower processing speed, difficulty following complex grammatical sentences and word retrieval difficulties also need to be considered.

The aim of assessing a person's general communication and cognitive ability is to help understand at what level to pitch the information required for decision making and which communication tools would be most helpful for that individual to aid with choice making.

The next step is to start conversations to support the individual to understand and communicate the information relevant to the specific question.

The level of the person's cognitive and communication ability will mean that conversations are tailored to the individual's needs, but it is useful to have a toolbox of strategies to choose from (see Table 8.1). For communication impaired clients, this decision making assessment should be ideally supported by an SLT and another familiar healthcare professional. The presence of family members is useful in terms of the client having a familiar person present but can become a challenge if the family member is not impartial or if there are mixed opinions within the family group.

Table 8.1 Some strategies and tools that can help to facilitate these conversations

Setup of conversa-tions	• Talk to the client's carers and arrange a time of day that is optimal for their best communication. For example, communication impairments tend to be worse with tiredness, so early morning, just after a meal or evening time are times to avoid. • Book a quiet room in advance. Hospital wards and nursing homes often have day rooms or family rooms that can be booked out. • Put a sign on the door to avoid interruptions. • Ensure you have a good knowledge of the client's receptive and expressive language ability from previous assessments and have had prior conversations to become familiar with their use of language or communication aids.
Practical preparations	• Check that the client is comfortable and is aware of the reason behind the assessment. • Check that hearing aids work and the person has their glasses, if required. • If the client uses electronic communication aids, make sure these are charged or have batteries.
Communi-cation tools	• Use any tools that can help to support understanding and that can be used to help the person express choices. Examples include the following: - Pictures - Photographs - Objects - Symbols - Alphabet charts - Pen and paper - Communication aids that are familiar to the client, including eye gaze systems. - Communication books.
Language style	• Language should be adapted to the level of receptive and expressive language found on assessment. • Present the information as clearly and simply as possible. • Avoid asking any leading questions. • Repeat keywords and phrases. • Allow processing time before expecting a response. • Write questions or keywords down to support understanding and processing. • Open questions produce high language demand for responding. Giving two or three choices can help to reduce the language load. Responses can be given verbally or by pointing to a written choice. • Ask the question more than once to check for consistency of responses. • Give alternative choices in a different order and check for consistency of response. • Repeat the client's response back to check that you have understood correctly. • Observe any non-verbal language and check for consistency of this response (e.g. nodding or shaking head, thumbs up or down and any signs of distress).
After assessment	• Document in the client's records. • Repeat the assessment another time to check retention of information. • If all measures to support the client's communication have been employed and there are inconsistent responses, or if the client is not able to understand or communicate the consequences of their choices, then it is deemed that they do not have cognitive ability to make this particular decision at this time and a best-interests decision is required.

Communication case example

Rosa, aged 85, is in an older person's rehabilitation hospital following a stroke. Staff are planning for her discharge from the hospital and feel she would be safer to be discharged to a care home where she would continue to receive 24-hour care. Rosa has been looking forward to returning home, where she previously lived independently, and appears to become distressed when a care home is mentioned. She has a communication impairment following her stroke, and staff have wondered whether she is able to make the decision about returning home or to a care home.

Communication ability: Assessment indicates that Rosa can understand and follow instructions at a two to three keyword level and responds well to written prompts of keywords to aid her understanding. She can make a choice with two written words by pointing to the correct word to respond to a simple question. She says very little verbally in response to questions, repeating (perseverating on) particular words when responding to a question. She is very expressive non-verbally, nodding or shaking her head and using facial expression. Photographs and pictures are also useful tools to help her understanding and for her to point to for expressing choice. She indicates her basic needs by pointing to an object or a picture in her communication book.

Specific decision for assessment: Can Rosa understand, retain and weigh up the information to clearly communicate an informed decision about her discharge destination?

Assessment: In order to make an informed decision about her discharge destination, Rosa needs to demonstrate that she understands and is aware of the consequences of accepting the risks of returning to her own home, including some risk of falls and not having care available 24 hours a day, rather than a care home where these risks will be reduced. She has been informed of the risks of returning home several times, so the assessment will also check for retention of this information. The assessment was carried out by an SLT and an OT.

As a first assessment, ten pictures were shown to her, depicting general dangerous situations (e.g. a toaster with a knife inside of it), and Rosa was asked to sort them in to categories of dangerous or not dangerous. She was consistently able to categorise these pictures correctly and demonstrate understanding of what is considered to be a dangerous situation.

Following on from this, she was presented with written choices – own home or care home – and given a selection of pictures to categorise under each. These included the risk of falls,

24-hour care and other functional items, such as meal preparation and toileting. Written and spoken keywords were used to help her understand the pictures.

Rosa was able to demonstrate that she understood the risks of returning home and consistently indicated this as her preference. However, she was unable to consistently demonstrate the consequences of the risks, such as being admitted to a hospital from a fall or only being able to have carers at certain times of the day. Therefore, at this time, she did not appear to have the full mental capacity to weigh up the consequences of her decision. This was demonstrated on three occasions.

Outcome: Rosa was clearly expressing a choice to go back to her own home. There was a discussion with her, her family and her healthcare professionals to decide what to do in her best interests. She had two visits home with the OT, and it became clearer to Rosa that returning home at this point would be difficult. A compromise was agreed between everyone that as her mobility and communication were improving, she would go to a care home as a temporary measure, with input from the Community Rehabilitation Team, and that the decision would be reviewed in four weeks' time.

Decision making and swallow impairment

People who have swallowing difficulties regularly have to consider options regarding the management of their symptoms. These decisions occur on a spectrum, from the recommendations of adapting or avoiding certain foods, to the decision to receive non-oral feeding (such as a feeding tube) when the swallow is not safe enough to meet nutritional needs orally without significant risk of aspiration pneumonia or choking.

SLTs are the principal clinicians to provide recommendations, based on a thorough swallow assessment, and will balance their recommendations to a client based on the presentation of their swallowing, risk factors for developing aspiration pneumonia and quality of life (see Chapter 7). That said, it remains the choice of the recipient of the advice to decide whether they want to adhere to these recommendations, and they need to make this decision with understanding of the risks involved in not following the recommendations. These risks include aspiration pneumonia, choking, increased risk of hospital admission and even death.

In some cases, a decline in swallowing can be predictable, with severe dysphagia being a common outcome of many of the progressive neurological disorders. This can allow the clinician to have frank but sensitive discussions with the client and family about their views on long-term feeding tubes in the event that the swallow becomes unsafe for any oral intake or the swallow is so poor that nutritional intake is compromised. This conversation ideally needs to take place whilst the person retains the mental capacity to understand and make such decision. The person can be offered the option of a formal, legal advanced care plan to refuse a feeding tube if they have strong feelings against this procedure, or they can sign a statement of wishes for or against a feeding tube, which would be taken into account in later discussions.

Dysphagia is common in older people but may occur with a less predictable pattern, given the heterogeneity of symptoms of ageing and different comorbidities. It can be a severe infection and hospital admission that tip the balance of the swallow into the category of unsafe. These episodes are difficult to predict and, therefore, plan for but can cause older person to temporarily lose the mental capacity to be able to be involved in discussions about management of their swallowing difficulty.

Whilst a formal discussion around management of swallowing impairments and wishes and preferences is likely to be held with people who have received a terminal diagnosis, this is much less common practice for older people in general unless they have prompted this themselves.

There are a variety of decisions that can be made as part of managing a swallowing impairment. Some of these are listed subsequently. As mentioned previously, if the person's ability to make the decision is in doubt, an assessment of mental capacity needs to take place with the person being given all practicable support to make the choice in question.

Examples of decisions to manage swallowing difficulties

- Avoiding certain foods.
- Modifying the texture of certain foods.
- Modifying the texture of fluids (e.g. making fluids thicker).
- Following strategies, such as head postures, when swallowing or pacing.
- Whether to have a short- or long-term feeding tube.

Advanced care planning when continuing oral intake with risk of aspiration

As mentioned in Chapter 7, there are circumstances in which a feeding tube might not be an option for an older person. This could be in the case of an advanced directive to refuse one or a current informed choice not to have one. It can also be the case that the person is not deemed medically suitable to have a feeding tube in circumstances where the risks outweigh the benefits.

In these cases, the person is likely to continue to have food and drink orally with a risk of developing aspiration pneumonia or choking. Such risk can be mitigated with excellent mouthcare and individualised swallowing advice from an SLT, but the risk will remain and the potential consequences discussed.

Advanced care planning needs to take place to decide how to manage any future episodes of aspiration pneumonia. For example, will antibiotic treatment be given? Will the person be admitted to the hospital? These plans should be documented and communicated clearly with relevant health professionals. Many services have their own guidelines or policies around continuing with to eat and drink orally with risk of choking or aspiration.

Swallowing Case Example

Gwen is a 74-year old with recently diagnosed motor neurone disease. She has had difficulty swallowing for about one year.

A diagnosis of motor neurone disease means that her swallow is likely to continue to deteriorate to the extent that her swallow will probably become unsafe to have food or drink orally, and there will be a high risk of choking, aspiration pneumonia and failure to meet nutritional requirements. As the swallow becomes less safe, a long-term feeding tube, such as a radiologically inserted gastrostomy (RIG) or a percutaneous endoscopic gastrostomy (PEG), is a treatment option to provide nutrition, hydration and medication, and to reduce the risk of aspiration pneumonia.

Communication ability: Gwen has mild-moderate dysarthria. She is able to communicate verbally, but her speech can become less intelligible when she is tired. She sometimes writes words down if she is having difficulty making herself understood.

Swallowing ability: Signs of oral and pharyngeal stage impairments. She has difficulty chewing foods due to oral-muscular weakness and coughs on drinks if drinking too quickly. Current recommendations from the speech and language therapist are IDDSI level 0 thin drinks and level 7 regular easy chew foods (see Appendix 1) with prompts to take time.

Discussion around feeding tubes: Gwen has researched her diagnosis and is aware that her swallowing will become more difficult and a feeding tube would be an option in future. A conversation takes place between Gwen, her consultant, her dietitian and her speech and language therapist. The likely risks of a deteriorating swallow are discussed as well as the potential risks of feeding tubes and their insertion.

There is no reason to doubt Gwen's mental capacity to state her advanced wishes around tube feeding. She is able to demonstrate verbally that she understands the advantages and disadvantages of each decision.

Outcome: Gwen decides that she will make an advanced statement of wishes against having a feeding tube at the time of her swallow becoming less safe. She decides against a legally binding advanced directive but wants her wishes and preferences to be documented.

However, her swallow continues to deteriorate, and she is admitted to the hospital on three occasions with aspiration pneumonia. Her advanced wishes around not having a feeding tube is revisited. Although her communication has also deteriorated, she is able to write down what she wants to say. At this time, Gwen indicates that she has changed her mind and would like a feeding tube but would like to continue with small amounts to eat orally for her quality of life. She is able to demonstrate that she understands the benefits and risks of her decision.

Chapter summary

- There are complex choices to consider in older age around matters such as care arrangements, health scenarios and finances.
- There are options of either formally or legally stating future wishes.
- The trajectory of decline is less clear in older people, which can make it difficult to know when to proceed with care planning discussions.
- Mental capacity assessment is required when a person's capacity to make a specific decision is in doubt.
- A communication impairment can make decision making more complex, and specific communication support is required.
- There are several considerations of management options and advanced care planning needs for older people with swallowing impairment.

References

Age UK (2021) *Advance Decisions (Living Wills) What Is an Advanced Statement?* www.ageuk.org.uk.

Jethwa, DP and Onalaja, O (2015) Advanced care planning and palliative medicine in dementia: A literature review. *BJPsych Bulletin*. 39: 74-78.

Mental Capacity Act (2005) www.legislation.gov.uk accessed 25/6/2021 at 13.41.

NHS Advanced Decision (Living Will) (2020) www.nhs.uk accessed 17/10/2020 at 9.41.

NHS Mental Capacity Act Information (2021) www.nhs.uk accessed 25/6/2021 at 13.06.

Poppe, M, Burleigh, S and Banerjee, S (2013) Qualitative Evaluation of Advanced Care Planning in Early Dementia. *PLOS One*. 8 (4).

Zuscak, SJ, Peisah, C and Ferguson, A (2015) A collaborative approach to supporting communication in the assessment of decision making capacity. *Disability and Rehabilitation*. 38 (11): 1107-1114.

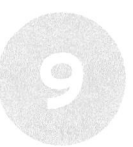

MANAGEMENT OF COMMUNICATION AND SWALLOWING AT THE END OF LIFE

DOI: 10.4324/9781003058090-10

Introduction to palliative and end of life care

Palliative and end of life care is integral to the work of healthcare professionals working with older people. Death most often occurs when people are in older age. Public Health England PHE (2019a) found that two-thirds of deaths in England in 2017 occurred in people who were 75 years old or above, and a third of these total deaths were people aged 90 years and older.

Death of friends, spouses or family is a more frequent occurrence in later life, with bereavement and loss a significant feature of older age. Thoughts of one's own death might feel more real in older age, especially if experiencing terminal illness or long-term ill health. Beliefs and attitudes towards death vary widely and tend to be very personal to an individual. Spiritual beliefs, cultural customs, personality type and life experience all influence how a person might feel about death.

Palliative and end of life care for older people crosses all settings. Statistics of those who died in older age indicate that 46% of people over 75 died in a hospital in England in 2017 (PHE, 2019b), and around 30% of people over 75 died in care homes (PHE, 2019a) among the most common causes of death in older age in 2017 were cancer, heart disease and pneumonia (PHE, 2019a). Frailty is also a leading cause of death in older people (British Geriatrics Society, 2020).

Palliative and end of life care

The World Health Organisation describes palliative care as care with the aims of improving quality of life for clients and the families of clients experiencing life-threatening illness, relieving pain and any other distressing symptoms, and addressing physical, psychological and spiritual needs.

Palliative care tends to begin at the stage when an illness becomes terminal. There may still be medical treatment, but this is done with the aim of relieving distressing symptoms rather than curing the disease. At the palliative care stage, plans can be made with the client and their family or friends about treatment options and preferences, attitudes towards death and opinions about place of death. Emotional support is also provided. Depending on the type of disease and the time of the diagnosis, people might spend many years receiving palliative care or just a short time.

End of life care forms a distinct part of palliative care, although the terms are sometimes used interchangeably. The Royal College of Nursing (2022) states that end of life care refers to approximately the last year of life but may also refer to the last months, weeks, days or hours of life, depending on the situation.

The dying stage may have been discussed and planned for earlier in the palliative care phase, especially with people who have a terminal diagnosis. However, the end of life stage can arrive more acutely; for example in the case of sudden serious infection or injury necessitating plans and discussions having to take place more urgently. Norton and Talerico (2000) note that although planning for end of life care is the gold standard, this often does not take place until late in the dying trajectory.

Palliative and end of life care is usually provided by a multidisciplinary team of professionals, each with expertise in supporting clients and their families and improving quality of life at the end of life. The British Geriatrics Society (2020) report that the best and most person-centred end of life care occurs when there is a multidisciplinary team holistically supporting clients and families.

Identifying palliative and end of life care needs in older people

Palliative and end of life care tends to focus on terminal illness. With some individual variation, these illnesses tend to follow patterns of deterioration, which can facilitate identification of when a person is entering the end of life stages.

It can be more difficult to identify when older people are at the stage when they need to receive palliative or end of life care. Lloyd et al. (2016) report that end of life trajectories for people in very old age or with frailty tend to be more prolonged and less acute and predictable than those with a diagnosis of terminal illness, such as cancer. Illness in older people can also present with different symptoms to those in younger people (see Chapter 1), and this, combined with changes to cognition and other comorbidities, can make end of life symptoms more of a challenge to predict.

Åvik Persson et al. (2018) report that older people in nursing homes tend to receive less adequate palliative care than younger people because of difficulty identifying when the stages of dying are beginning.

Nonetheless, older people have a right to high-quality, interdisciplinary care to support them to have optimal quality of life and comfort as they move into their final stages of life. End of life care should always focus on the person as an individual, with tailored treatment to maximise comfort.

Communication and swallowing difficulties are common at the end of life. Speech and language therapists (SLTs) are an invaluable resource in the multidisciplinary team supporting people at the end of their life (Pollens, 2004). They can assess and advise to facilitate effective communication between the client, family members and healthcare staff, and use their expertise to advise on eating, drinking and swallowing at the end of life. This chapter discusses management of communication and eating, drinking and swallowing difficulties at the end of life.

As much of the previous chapter addressed decisions that tend to occur as part of the palliative care; this chapter will focus on communication and swallowing difficulties in the last few weeks, days and hours of life.

Communication at the end of life

The need to be able to engage in good quality communication with others is vital when caring for people who are dying. The needs of each person at this stage will be unique, and although it can be planned for to a certain extent, it is impossible to fully predict how the dying person will feel at this stage or what emotions will come up for their family or friends. People who are dying may express a wish to talk to certain people or bring up important topics that they would like to talk about, and these communication requests need to be supported as much as possible. Other people might withdraw and have little interest in talking.

It is important to talk to the person about the fact that they are dying. It has been found that conversations with elderly people about their imminent death occur less frequently than with younger people (Lindskog et al., 2015). Unless people have previously specifically stated that they do not want to know, it is good practice to initiate these conversations to help support the person emotionally and to help meet any needs or requests for their final stage of life. Having the conversation about death paves the way for the person to be involved in decision making about their own death and to have some sense of control about how they would like that to be; for example, preference to die at home or the hospital, or choices regarding medication. Some of these decisions may have been made previously in formal advanced care plans (see Chapter 8), but these can be revisited or adapted if the person has retained mental capacity and appears to have changed their opinion. Otherwise, family members with legal power to make medical decisions, if the person has lost mental capacity, can be consulted to help with decision making.

The experience and comfort of clinicians in explicitly bringing up the topic of dying has been associated with client satisfaction at this stage (Norton and Talerico, 2000). Therefore, clinicians who are new to working with dying clients would benefit from observing their more experienced colleagues having these conversations to help them to feel more comfortable and prepared for their own similar conversations. These conversations need to respect the cultural and spiritual beliefs of the dying person. Any familiar healthcare professional can have these conversations with the client and their family or friends. People with a communication impairment are likely to require extra support from an SLT to facilitate understanding of the conversation and to support them to make responses or decisions.

Communication impairments

Communication impairments are associated with several of the terminal illnesses, including progressive neurological diseases, such as motor neurone disease, dementia and advanced head and neck cancer. With progressive neurological disease, such as motor neurone disease, speech will often be unintelligible at the end of life stage. People who have dementia will often have severely reduced communication ability towards the end of life but will usually still show some signs of non-verbal communication, such as feeling pain or needing comfort (Alzheimer's Society, 2021).

Symptoms brought about by the dying process can result in exacerbation of these existing communication impairments or bring about new communication difficulties in a client who did not previously have an impairment (see Table 9.1). For example, some side effects of medications used at the end of life can cause drowsiness and more effortful speech. Some of these communication difficulties can be planned for, but there will be variability in the severity of symptoms and how these impact on communication ability. This is particularly the case if the person has a pre-existing communication disorder because of their illness or a previous stroke, head injury or learning difficulty.

Table 9.1   Some of the symptoms affecting communication during the end of life stage

End of life symptoms that can impact on communication ability
Agitation and restlessness
Anxiety and/or depression
Pain
Fatigue
Confusion
Dry mouth
Sore mouth
Withdrawal
Difficulty managing saliva

It might be difficult for older people to communicate these symptoms in the dying phase. It has been found that elderly people are less likely to be assessed for severity of pain at end of life compared to their younger counterparts (Lindskog et al., 2015). This may be because they are not communicating their pain in the same way or that healthcare professionals had not recognised the end of life stage and the symptoms that might occur alongside.

Given the fact that people who are actively dying might have difficulty communicating their needs verbally, it is important to have caregivers who are sensitive to non-verbal language. SLTs will be skilled in carrying out communication assessments of both non-verbal and verbal language and giving individualised advice as part of the multidisciplinary team (Pollens, 2004). Family and friends who know the person well will also be able to support with identifying non-verbal signals.

There are various ways a clinician might work to facilitate communication at this time.

Examples of communication work at the end of life include the following:

- Establishing an effective communication method to help with communication of the level of pain and need for pain medication. Pain can be assessed by using rating scales, picture choices or observation of non-verbal signals.
- Observing and documenting non-verbal language. For example, does the person appear to be comforted by touch? Do facial expressions or vocalisations change with distress or discomfort? Does the person appear to indicate thirst or hunger or fatigue?
- Ensuring that all communication tools and assistive technology is up to date. Older people with pre-existing communication difficulties may have access to these, such as eye gaze systems, iPads and picture communication books. Check that the client, family members and other healthcare professionals know how these are used for communication.
- Supporting the client to be able to have conversations that are important to them. A person might wish to make amends with a family member, have significant conversations with children or grandchildren or communicate their feelings of love and affection or words of wisdom. Create time for these conversations, provide picture resources or support the client to dictate a letter.
- Giving strategies to family and healthcare staff to facilitate communication.

Clients may also have particular goals related to communication at the end of life, and these need to be discussed and supported. For example, a person might want to write or dictate a letter or record a video. Other clients may not wish to interact much but are comforted by a short phone message from a friend or family member.

In the 'Resources' section at the end of this chapter, there is a leaflet for families and/or carers to explain how to support communication at the end of life.

Eating and drinking and swallowing at the end of life

The desire to eat and drink diminishes when people are dying. The body does not seem to require or metabolise food and drink in the same way. This can be a particularly distressing symptom for relatives and friends caring for the person, as it is obvious that they are not receiving enough nutrition or hydration. In some cultures, the giving of nourishing food and drink is a significant caring behaviour when people are ill, and so for some, it can feel as though their relative is not being cared for well enough if they are not able to give them adequate food or drink, or that they are contributing to their death by not providing these.

Swallowing difficulties (dysphagia) are very common in terminal illnesses. There is overlap in the terminal illnesses, which have both communication impairment and swallow impairment as symptoms, such as progressive neurological diseases, dementia and advanced head and neck cancer. Dysphagia will present at various times during the disease trajectory but will become progressively worse as the disease progresses and towards the end of life. Some people with these illnesses will have chosen to have a long-term feeding tube, such as a PEG (percutaneous endoscopic gastrostomy), as their swallowing worsened in earlier stages of the disease process.

As previously mentioned, it can be difficult to judge when older people without a terminal diagnosis are entering the end phase of life. Some medical professionals use decline in swallowing as a potential signal for decline into end of life. However, older people in hospital can become confused and anxious by a change in environment or routine, which can lead to a temporarily reduced swallowing ability and loss of appetite, or their swallow could be decompensated by an infection but is not a signal that they are dying. People with dementia can experience swallowing difficulties as a terminal symptom, but they can also experience swallowing difficulties much earlier in the disease, depending on the type of dementia or comorbidities they might have. These overlapping symptoms can make it a

Table 9.2   Some of the terminal symptoms associated with eating, drinking and swallowing

End of life symptoms that can impact on swallowing ability
Difficulty managing saliva
Reduced reflexive swallow might lead to saliva not being swallowed automatically and, therefore, accumulating in the mouth
Retention of saliva or secretions in the throat and difficulty clearing these
Thick secretions in the mouth and throat
Dry mouth
Sore mouth
Reduced desire to eat and drink
Coughing on food or drink
Difficulty swallowing medication
Difficulty coordinating the cycle of swallowing and breathing due to shortness of breath
Fatigue

challenge to discern whether the older client with swallowing difficulties is indeed at the end of life.

However, it is important that this is judged correctly as the reduced appetite or swallowing difficulties may be reversed if treatment is given in some circumstances. The end of life decision based on poor appetite or swallowing difficulties should take place after a considered multidisciplinary team decision along with discussion with the client, if possible, or family members and needs to include observation of all symptoms, acute or chronic onset of symptoms, client's previous wishes about treatment and responsiveness to treatment.

As with communication difficulties, swallowing difficulties associated with the terminal illness can be exacerbated at the end of life, or symptoms associated with the dying process can bring about eating, drinking and swallowing difficulties (see Table 9.2).

It is important to mention that these symptoms can occur earlier in many of the progressive diseases, such as dementia or motor neurone disease, so these need to be taken in context and may not necessarily indicate end of life.

Assessment and management of swallowing difficulties at the end of life

The assessment of a person's swallow at the end of life should be sensitive to the current circumstances. For example, an objective assessment, such as a videofluoroscopy, is likely to cause more disruption and discomfort for a client at this stage. It is also unlikely to add anything useful in terms of management unless there is a specific symptom that is distressing for a client and cannot be detected or alleviated via strategies from a bedside swallow assessment.

It is unlikely that a new feeding tube or a decision to place a feeding tube would be made if a person is thought to be at the end of their life, as it is unlikely to make any difference to the outcome. It is likely that the person will be at increased risk of aspiration pneumonia and choking at this stage. This risk needs to be explained to the person and family members, and mitigated for as much as possible by way of alleviating any distressing symptoms whilst maintaining comfort, choice and dignity.

There might be certain textures of food and drink that could reduce the risk of aspiration and/or choking. Modifying textures of food or fluid can help to reduce the risk of choking and any distressing symptoms associated with aspiration, such as coughing on swallowing. Food that is softer or easier to chew can reduce the effort of chewing and the risk of choking. Drinks that are naturally thick, such as milkshakes or made thicker with thickening powder, may be easier to swallow and reduce some of the distressing symptoms of coughing.

Modifying food and drink should be based on a swallow assessment by a speech and language therapist to identify the consistencies that would be of most benefit to the individual. Some people welcome these consistency changes to alleviate the effort of chewing and the aspiration symptoms. Other people do not like the consistency changes and would prefer to accept an increased risk of aspiration or choking on food and drink that is not modified.

Other examples of managing eating, drinking and swallowing at the end of life include the following:

- Working with the client to find out what they would like in terms of oral intake.
- Optimising good mouth care for comfort and to reduce soreness and dryness of mouth.
- Working with the medical team to manage difficult secretions to optimise comfort.
- Working with the client and family to establish a care plan based on favourite tastes or flavours.
- Reducing any distressing symptoms associated with swallowing with advice on upright positioning, pace of feeding and texture modification of food or drinks.
- Explaining to family members or multidisciplinary team about swallowing symptoms and giving advice and strategies.

The person might have particular goals, such as tasting a food that brings comfort, or there may be specific requests for refreshing items, such as ice cream. At this point in time, the nutritional content of the food or drink is not an issue, so it does not matter if the food is not nutritionally balanced.

In the 'Resources' section at the end of this chapter, there is a leaflet for families and/or carers to explain how to support eating, drinking and swallowing at the end of life.

End of life care plans

An end of life care plan is a useful tool to communicate the communication and swallowing needs of a dying client to family members and medical or caring staff involved in the care. The document needs to be individualised to the needs of the client and flexible enough to be changed regularly to accommodate changing symptoms during this time. A copy can be placed near the person's bed with their consent or their families' consent, if the client is unable, and a copy for the notes. At the end of the chapter, there is a proforma for an end of life care plan.

After the death of a client

In the weeks following the death of a client, it is good practice for a clinician who was closely involved to contact their family or close friend to pass on condolences and hear about their experiences. This needs to be judged sensitively, taking into account the nature of the grieving process and how closely the healthcare professional worked with the family.

It can be a time of reflecting on service provision in terms of support for the client's communication and swallowing at the end of life, how supported the family or friend felt during this process and whether they feel anything could have been done differently to improve the service.

Working with people who are dying requires significant emotional resources on behalf of the healthcare professional. The clinician may have worked with the dying person for some time and developed a strong working relationship. They may have had to support their client to communicate a difficult topic at the end of life. They may also feel that they could have done more than they were able to. It is important that the healthcare professional can access adequate support if required. This can take the form of reflection and debrief with colleagues as well as dedicated managerial support.

Chapter summary

- It can be difficult to predict when an older person is dying, particularly when they do not have a terminal illness.
- End of life care in older people needs to be person centred and ideally managed by a specialist multidisciplinary team.
- New communication and swallowing difficulties can arise at the end of life as well as exacerbation of existing ones.
- Speech and language therapists have specialist skills to improve the comfort and quality of life for older people who are dying.

Case examples

Case example 1

Background: Charles is an 89-year-old with dementia. He lives in a care home and has a history of recurrent chest infections over the last three months. Following a swallowing assessment, he was advised to have IDDSI level 2 mildly thick drinks (see Appendix 1) to reduce his risk of aspiration, but his swallowing has deteriorated, and he is coughing on the thickened fluids and food. He has been admitted to the hospital twice in the last month with pneumonia and now has another severe chest infection. Each time he gets admitted to the hospital, he becomes agitated and anxious with the unfamiliar environment and staff. Despite antibiotics, he continues to have a fever and is having difficulty clearing secretions from his throat.

Staff at the care home and his GP feel he might be at the end of his life. They request a swallowing assessment for advice and support. He has formal documentation, which he organised at the time of his dementia diagnosis, that documents refusal of feeding tubes in the event of him being unable to eat and drink orally as a result of his dementia.

His communication is now very limited for conversations in the present, but he does like to talk about his memories of holidays.

Swallow assessment: A swallow assessment is carried out by a speech and language therapist at the care home. The swallow assessment indicates that Charles appears to be at risk of aspiration on all oral intake and, therefore, at increased risk of aspiration pneumonia. He appears to enjoy small amounts of IDDSI level 4 pureed food, especially puddings, and he is accepting of IDDSI level 2 mildly thick fluids. However, he has a tendency to reach for the water jug but will not drink thickened water. He does not appear to be distressed by his aspiration symptoms.

End of life conversation: Charles was not able to participate in the discussion, but his non-verbal behaviours were acknowledged and considered. His daughter joined by video call, and his doctor and SLT were in attendance. It was decided that it was not in Charles's best interests to be admitted to hospital again due to the apparent distress this causes him and due to the irreversible nature of his chest infections. He previously set out in a formal, legal document that he did not want a feeding tube. It was decided to continue to offer him oral intake, making it as safe as possible with advice on sitting upright for oral intake, doing regular mouth care and using texture modification, but allowing him to have sips of unthickened water for his quality of life and comfort. Increased risk of aspiration pneumonia was acknowledged and documented.

Case example 2

Background: Dorothy is 98 years old. She has been admitted to the hospital with a chest infection. She has a history of recurrent chest and urinary tract infections over the last six months. Staff at her care home report poor appetite and weight loss recently. She moved to her care home ten years ago following a stroke. Her language was affected by her stroke, and as a result, she is unable to understand complex sentences and has significant word finding difficulties. Many years ago, prior to the stroke, she had mentioned to family that she would not want to be resuscitated if she was very unwell, but she does not have any formal documentation for this and no discussion on this topic has taken place since her stroke.

Current presentation: In the hospital, she has been sleeping much of the time and eating and drinking very little, and her infection has not responded to medication. She waves staff away when they bring her food or drink or medication and appears reluctant to engage in any conversation. The multidisciplinary team in hospital feel that she might be nearing the end of her life and would like to engage Dorothy in this discussion as much as possible. They request a communication assessment from Speech and Language Therapy due to her language impairment.

Communication assessment: Communication assessment was carried out by an SLT. Fatigue, pain and poor attention were barriers to a full assessment. Assessment was carried out in separate shorter periods rather than all at once in view of these barriers. Assessment indicated that Dorothy could understand simple yes or no closed questions, but her answers needed to be checked for consistency of her responses. She was able to indicate some of her needs by pointing to objects around her or to parts of her body. She could use a rating scale to indicate pain or discomfort and could also read and understand single keyword instructions.

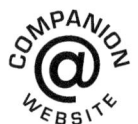

End of life conversation: Conversation about end of life took place with Dorothy, an SLT and a doctor, with family present for some of the conversations. Conversations happened over two days, with short conversations of around ten minutes each. Keywords were written down to aid Dorothy's understanding and retention of information. Dorothy indicated that she did not want to try any more medication and consistently said yes when asked if she knew she was at the end of her life. She indicated from a written multiple choice of hospital or care home that she wanted to die in her care home. Dorothy's family were informed of these conversations.

End of life care decision: It was decided that Dorothy would go back to her care home to die as soon as they were able to accept her. She had become drowsier and was eating very little. An end of life care plan for her communication and swallowing was started in the hospital based on Dorothy's current presentation (see next section) and sent to the care home for staff to amend as required.

Resources

- End of life care plan
- Example of a completed end of life care plan using information from case example 2
- Supporting communication needs at the end of life: Information for family and friends
- Eating, drinking and swallowing at the end of life: Leaflet for family and friends

End of life care plans

Table 9.3 End of life care plans

Name: DOB: Name and contact number of clinician completing form: Name and contact number of significant family member / friend:
Communication   Communication of pain or distress: Communication of basic needs (e.g. thirst and discomfort):   Communication in conversation: Other: **Swallowing**   Frequency of mouthcare: Secretion management: Frequency of oral intake: Textures/modifications of food or drink: Favourite flavours: Other:

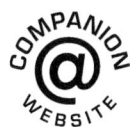

Example of a completed end of life care plan using information from case example 2

Table 9.4 Completed end of life care plan

Name: *Dorothy* **DOB:** **Name and contact number of clinician completing form:** **Name and contact number of significant family member / friend:**
Communication **Communication of pain or distress:** Dorothy appears to communicate pain by becoming agitated and restless in bed. She will often try to pull the bed covers off. She appears more settled after administration of pain medication. She can sometimes demonstrate her level of pain using a picture rating scale. **Communication of basic needs (e.g. thirst and discomfort):** She will point to a cup of water at times to indicate thirst. She tends to shut her mouth when she does not want any more food. She will sometimes try to rearrange her pillows, indicating discomfort. **Communication in conversation:** Dorothy is sleeping most of the time but has periods when she is more alert. She becomes tired easily so is better with short conversations. Important conversations should be kept short and repeated later on to check Dorothy's understanding and to help her process what is being said. She will say when she wants to be left alone or wave people away. **Other:** Dorothy likes to have a photo of her dog, Ben, by her bedside so she can always see him. Her family visit regularly and look through photographs with her. **Swallowing** **Frequency of mouthcare:** Four times a day. Check that Dorothy's mouth and lips are clean and moist and not sore. **Secretion management:** No invasive suctioning techniques. She may require suctioning of secretions from the front of her mouth. Speak to medical team for appropriate medication if secretions are becoming distressing or Dorothy is unable to clear them. **Frequency of oral intake:** Offer food and drink regularly throughout the day. **Textures/modifications of food or drink:** Food: Dorothy is only eating ice cream, mousse or yoghurt now, so offer her these regularly throughout the day. She will sometimes have a few spoons of mashed potato with cheese at mealtimes. Drink: Dorothy is coughing sometimes when drinking. She is drinking water and occasional cups of tea. Please ensure she is sitting as upright as possible when drinking and has small sips, one at a time, to reduce any distressing symptoms of aspiration. **Favourite flavours:** Vanilla or strawberry. **Other:** Dorothy prefers to use a teaspoon rather than a larger spoon when eating.

Supporting communication needs at the end of life: Information for family and friends

Towards the end of life, people may not be able to communicate as effectively or in the same way as before. This can be difficult for close relatives and friends to observe, and it is sometimes hard to know what to do and how to communicate in this situation.

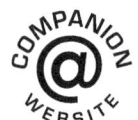

This leaflet is designed to help you understand how communication might change towards the end of life and give ideas for what you can do support your relative or friend.

How communication can change towards the end of life

- Some often find speaking or interacting with other people more effortful and tiring.
- People might experience a sore or dry mouth.
- The person's speech might become more difficult to understand.
- They may have more difficulty understanding what is being said or following a conversation.
- Some people might have symptoms, such as confusion, or restlessness that can make conversation more challenging.
- Some people might withdraw and not show interest in talking.
- Some people want to discuss important topics before they die.

What you can do to support communication at the end of life

- Talk about topics that you know your relative/friend enjoys hearing about.
- Try not to avoid difficult or emotional topics. Give space and time for these. Ask your friend/relative to signal if they want the conversation to stop.
- Pause and leave space for them to reply or talk, but be aware that they may not. Sometimes they might just want to listen.
- Try to have shorter interactions to reduce fatigue levels.
- Observe whether there are certain times of the day when it is easier to have a conversation.
- Look for non-verbal clues that the person is ready for the interaction to finish (e.g. tiredness, poor concentration and restlessness).
- Consider that sometimes your relative/friend might want to just be with you rather than talk.
- Touch, such as hand-holding, can be a comfort for some people at the end of life.
- Play music that you know they enjoy or appear to be comforted by.
- Make the environment as calming as possible with familiar clothing, bedding and photographs.
- Talk about memories.
- Have an exercise book present to make a note of observations for other visitors (e.g. topics of conversation) and observation of non-verbal communication.
- Try pictures or ask closed questions to help understand specifically what is needed if a person is struggling to express their needs (e.g. 'Are you in pain?' and 'Is the pain in your legs?').

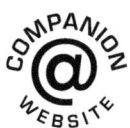

If your friend or relative is distressed by not being able to communicate their needs or if you need communication support to discuss difficult topics, please request a referral to a speech and language therapist (SLT). SLTs will be able to assess communication and provide individual communication strategies and support.

Eating, drinking and swallowing at the end of life: Leaflet for family and friends

Towards the end of life, eating and drinking habits are likely to change. This might be a gradual process or can happen more suddenly. The body tends not to need food and drink in the same way, and difficulties with swallowing can occur. Eating and drinking is a significant part of life, and giving comforting food to people when they are ill is often felt to be an act of caring. However, eating and drinking becomes less important when someone is in the last few weeks or days of life, and this can be difficult for friends and relatives to observe.

This leaflet is designed to give advice on what to expect with eating, drinking and swallowing towards the end of life, and give information on what you can do to make your loved one more comfortable.

How eating, drinking and swallowing can change towards the end of life

- Process of eating and drinking can be tiring and effortful.
- Side effects from medication can make people more sleepy and less able to eat.
- Effects, such as a dry or sore mouth, make eating and drinking uncomfortable.
- Loss of appetite.
- Changes to taste sensation.
- Difficulty chewing
- Coughing when swallowing
- Excess or thick secretions in the chest, throat or mouth.

What you can do to help

- Be aware that loss of appetite is normal towards the end of life and nutrition is less essential.
- Try softer, smoother types of food since chewing might be more of an effort.
- Offer regular sips of fluids. Ice lollies can also help to moisten the mouth.
- Offer small tastes of favourite flavours.
- Ensure your relative/friend is sitting as upright as possible if having anything to eat or drink.

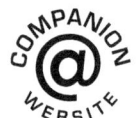

- Give regular mouthcare with gentle brushing and removal of any dry skin or secretions to improve comfort. A nurse or speech and language therapist can advise you on specific mouthcare.
- Ask the doctor for support if their mouth is dry or sore.
- Ask the doctor for support if there is difficulty managing saliva.
- Please request a swallow assessment and advice from a speech and language therapist if there are symptoms of coughing or choking when eating or drinking.

References

Alzheimer's Society (2021) End of life care: communication and physical needs www.alzheimers.org.uk accessed 24/4/22 at 14.07.

Åvik Persson, H et al. (2018) Early and late signs that precede dying among older persons in nursing homes: The multidisciplinary team's perspective. *BMC Geriatrics*. 18: 134.

British Geriatrics Society (2020) *End of Life Care in Frailty: Identification and Prognostication.* www.bgs.org.uk/resources/end-of-life-care-in-frailty-identification-and-prognostication accessed 7/11/2020 at 14.50

Lindskog, M, Tavelin, B and Lündstrom, S (2015) Old age as a risk factor for poor end of life care quality- a population based study of cancer deaths from the Swedish register of palliative care. *European Journal of Cancer*. 51 (10): 1331-1339.

Lloyd, A et al. (2016) Physical, social, psychological and existential trajectories of loss and adaptation towards the end of life for older people living with frailty: A serial interview study. *BMC Geriatrics*. 16 (1): 176.

Morley, JE (2004) A brief history of geriatrics. The Journals of Gerontology :Series A, volume 59. Issue 11

Norton, SA and Talerico, KA (2000) Facilitating end of life decision making strategies for communicating and assessing. *Journal of Gerontological Nursing*. 26 (9): 6-13.

Pollens, R (2004) Roles of speech and language pathologist in hospice care. *Journal of Palliative Medicine*. 7 (5).

Public Health England (2019a) *Deaths in People Aged 75 Years and Older in England in 2017*. www.gov.uk accessed 7/10/2020 at 10.20.

Public Health England (2019b) *Older People Who Died in Hospital: England 2017*. www.gov.uk accessed 21/5/2021 at 10.15.

Royal College of Nursing (2022) End of Life Care https://www.rcn.org.uk/clinical-topics/end-of-life-care accessed 24/4/22 at 13.56.

REFLECTING BACK AND LOOKING FORWARD TO THE FUTURE OF HEALTHCARE PROVISION FOR OLDER ADULTS

DOI: 10.4324/9781003058090-11

Section 1: Introduction

In the closing chapter of this book, we revisit and summarise the themes and the key learning points. Using our current knowledge about communication and swallowing impairments in older age, we look forward to how this knowledge can influence design of health and social care services to lead to better outcomes for older people in terms of living well in older age.

Section 2: Summary of themes and learning points

This book has journeyed through several topics aligned to the care of older people with communication and swallowing difficulties. The first chapters focused on foundation, prerequisite knowledge of the context of ageing in current society, physiology of ageing and special considerations for an older client group. The middle chapters discussed the evidence and theory behind communication and swallow impairments in older age, and the practical application of this knowledge in clinical settings. The final chapters addressed decision making and palliative and end of life care, which are integral to the work of all clinicians who are working with older people. The themes of these three sections of the book are discussed subsequently.

Ageing: society, physiology and rehabilitation

The early chapters of the book focus on framing the ageing process within the context of change from middle to old age. There has been a trend towards people living longer, although increased morbidity and chronic conditions means that many people are not necessarily living well, with good quality of life in their older years.

Feelings of loneliness are common in older age. These feelings can have a negative impact on physical health outcomes, including an increased risk of heart disease and stroke.

Older people have been particularly hit by the COVID-19 pandemic, both disproportionately in the rates of death and severe illness, and with being socially isolated.

Ageing has an inevitable effect on the physiology of the body, with brain atrophy, cognitive decline, and reduced muscle bulk and strength being of the most prominent changes. The body becomes less able to deal with stressors, such as infection or injury, and there is increased risk of developing frailty.

However, the speed at which the body ages and the severity of the impact of ageing on daily life affect everyone differently. To some extent, this can be determined by genetic predisposition, but there are lifestyle factors that also influence the impact of ageing. Overall fitness and muscle strength, the quality of social connections, cognitively stimulating activity, socio-economic status and nutritional intake are all associated with how much ageing impacts on the body and subsequent quality of life.

A good reserve of physical and cognitive fitness is a protective factor against the effects of ageing.

Neuroplasticity and rehabilitation potential continues throughout the lifespan, particularly if there is a good physical and cognitive reserve as a baseline. Older people can learn new skills but may be slower to acquire these or have more difficulty generalising the skills into different scenarios.

Age should never be a barrier to receiving high-quality, person-centred care. Older adults require access to assessment and intervention in the same way as their younger counterparts, but they may have different goals and different needs. Attitudes towards age and elderspeak are amongst the barriers to an effective working relationship with older people.

Communication and swallowing impairment in older age

The middle chapters of the book focused on changes to communication and swallowing in older age.

The ability to communicate effectively in later life can be affected in multiple ways with changes to technology, lifestyle factors leading to changing communication networks and psychological changes. The physiology of ageing impacts on several aspects of communication, from visual and hearing changes, changes to voice quality, word finding difficulties, slower processing speed and difficulty understanding complex grammatical sentences.

The eating, drinking and swallowing process is affected by reduced appetite, lifestyle changes and changes to dentition. Physiologically, there are changes to each of the phases of swallowing with sarcopenia, slowness of movement and diminished sensory signals impacting on the strength and safety of the swallow.

Perhaps frustratingly for clinicians, there can be little normative quantitative data on how much age impacts communication and swallowing. Ageing occurs on a spectrum, and the heterogeneity of this makes it difficult to provide a comparison with younger people in definitive terms. There is a delicate balance in which the normal changes of age can easily tip over into a disorder, which then has a significant impact on quality of life and functioning.

This is particularly the case with swallowing in that an older swallow is vulnerable to becoming disordered if there is an infection or a trauma in the body.

A speech and language therapist needs to take a thorough case history and assessment of the communication and/or swallowing impairment, to be aware of symptoms that might indicate an underlying disorder or a differential diagnosis and to action any onward referrals required. Any Speech and Language Therapy intervention needs to take into quality of life and person-centred goals.

Decision making and palliative care

The final section of the book discusses planning for the future and care at the end of life. Older adults need to be engaged in discussions about care planning and their wishes for the future, and to know the options of the decisions on offer to them. If they do not wish to make a legal refusal for certain treatments, they can be supported to make a statement of wishes. These conversations require a proactive approach and not waiting until a crisis of illness or hospital admission during which an older person might lose the ability to have full involvement in the discussions.

Some people will not want to make early decisions and prefer to go along with life as it happens. Of course, this is their preferred option, but it can be beneficial to bring up the conversation from time to time.

People with communication difficulties require support from SLTs to facilitate their ability to understand the information pertaining to decisions and to communicate their responses.

Palliative care has a strong tradition in clinical fields, such as cancer and progressive neurological illness, in which the trajectory of dying is more predictable. Dying as a result of older age can be more difficult to predict even if the person is very unwell, as the symptoms may present differently or in a vaguer fashion. This can mean that older people do not have access to the same quality of palliative or end of life care.

Learning outcomes

After reading this book, the key learning outcomes for clinicians are as follows:

- Knowledge of how natural ageing affects the physiology of the body and factors that influence this process. The difference between sarcopenia and frailty, and how these impact on an ageing body.

- Ability to consider the needs of an older client group and flexibly adapt to meet an older client's needs.

- Ability to identify aspects of normal ageing with regard to communication and swallowing and recognise the symptoms of an underlying pathological communication or swallowing disorder.

- Ability to use the toolkit of information sheets, strategies and exercises, and select appropriate ones to use with clients who have communication and/or swallow impairment and their families or carers.

- Awareness of the decision making processes in later life and of the need for clinicians to operate within a legal framework and to be able to support specific decision making with people who have communication and swallowing difficulties.

- Knowledge of how communication and swallowing can present at the end of life and how to manage these to promote comfort, reduce distress and contribute to a better quality of death.

Overall summary

Perhaps the overall message of the book is that ageing is inevitable but affects everyone individually. Older age has positive aspects and can bring about new opportunities, but many people also live less well with reduced quality of life in their later years.

The information in this book has taught us that ageing does not just affect one aspect of a person, and each older person requires treating holistically, from the level of the impairment through to their lifestyle factors. A word finding difficulty as a normal age-related change can become worse with low mood or reduced social interaction. A severe age-related swallow disorder is part of a bigger picture often including reduced nutritional intake and sarcopenia.

In the author's experience, the older client group has sometimes been viewed as a less attractive area to work in, with more focus on function-based care and support with ageing effects, clients declining into palliative care and less dramatic results from rehabilitation.

However, it is also the author's experience that this is an exciting field to work in. Working with older people requires innovation, flexibility and creativity. It is a privilege to work jointly with our older clients on setting goals to improve their wellbeing and functional ability at an important time of life.

Using evidence and knowledge of the factors influencing the impact of ageing, and the need for better quality palliative and end of life care for older people, we can see how services for older people could be transformed in future. This is discussed in the following section.

Section 3: The future of healthcare services for older adults

In recent years, there has been a battle to reduce the increasing number of older people admitted to hospital in crisis of illness or social need. This is partially because the infrastructure to provide quality health and social care for older people has not grown at the same rate as the number of people living into older age. This has led to a situation where efforts are focused on crisis management without the resources to address the bigger picture.

However, the increasing awareness of the factors for reducing the effects of ageing and the ability to assess individual risk factors for more significant ageing has led to the beginnings of transformation for services to take an early and more targeted approach to lessen the impact of ageing.

Transformation of healthcare for older adults could include the following aspects: education, screening, early intervention, palliative care and client involvement. These are detailed subsequently:

Education

Many people recognise signs of ageing, such as changes to skin, hair, hearing and sight. Other signs, such as muscle weakness and slower processing time, might not be so well recognised. Changes to communication and eating, drinking and swallowing might be even less well known.

On the one hand, it is good to educate people on the inevitable changes that age brings, to normalise these so that there is understanding and acceptance. Adaptations can then be made to enable older people to be able to fully participate in life despite ageing effects.

On the other hand, people need to know that whilst ageing is inevitable, the speed and severity of ageing can be somewhat reduced through lifestyle factors. This education needs to be directed at all age groups, as people can build up physical and cognitive reserve throughout their lives, and this will benefit them in later life. It is acknowledged that it can be difficult for younger people to imagine themselves in older age and to use this as a motivation to alter their lifestyle habits. Fortunately, healthy living messaging is widespread, and most people have some awareness of healthier lifestyle factors, although some people require more support to put these into action.

There has been increasing awareness of the benefits of exercise, social interaction and cognitively stimulating activities for older people with dedicated exercise groups, friendship groups and hobby groups. It is hoped that these will once more be in regular use as the COVID-19 pandemic subsides. As mentioned in Chapter 1, social prescribing can help vulnerable older people to access exercise and social groups.

As people in later life are at higher risk of developing disease, it is also necessary that they are educated to recognise suspicious symptoms early. There are already information messages about recognising stroke symptoms and symptoms of some cancers. There is a strong argument for spotting the symptoms of other conditions, such as frailty, which significantly impacts on quality of life in older age and can be more easily reversed in its early stages.

Awareness also needs to be raised that older people might present with different symptoms to those of younger people experiencing the same disease, so education is required to look out for signs, such as general malaise or confusion. Older people need prompting to visit their doctor if the side effects of their medication are negatively influencing their overall functioning and wellbeing.

Resources for education and monitoring of older adults in the community can be piloted, measured and researched for effectiveness in order to inform commissioning services and future service development.

Screening

The risk factors for significant ageing effects are known and can be used as part of a screening programme to identify which individuals are more at risk.

The prognostic indicators checklist in Chapter 2 is one informal example that can help triage which individuals need quicker access to assessment and intervention. However, this one is designed to give to clients after referral to triage how quickly an appointment is needed.

A wider, earlier screening programme is required to identify people as they go into older age to target people who might benefit from social prescribing or early intervention.

In the UK, general practitioners screen patients for frailty, as do community geriatricians. This is welcome and can help to predict who might require more support to reduce or prevent the decline into frailty. However, many of the formal frailty screens do not include questions about swallowing difficulty, which is one of the precursors to developing frailty (see Chapter 6). Maher et al. (2019) studied the benefit of a dysphagia screen as part of a frailty assessment and found that this was a reliable method of identifying dysphagia and those at risk of dysphagia.

Early intervention

Early intervention with older adults showing risk factors for significant ageing effects or frailty is key. Intervention at an early stage allows an older person to develop a greater reserve to mitigate later age-related decline and to reduce the risk of deteriorating function to a state that is less reversible.

The multifaceted nature of ageing and knowledge of potential protective factors gives a strong argument for dedicated interdisciplinary teams to provide early intervention, support and rehabilitation for older people. At present, rehabilitation teams often comprise only of Physiotherapy and Occupational Therapy, but with the often debilitating impact of communication and swallowing impairments in older age, it is essential that SLTs are integrated members of these teams, as well as dietitians who can provide nutritional support. There is evidence that muscle strength training can help delay or reverse frailty (Travers et al., 2019), but muscle strength training cannot be effective if there is an undiagnosed swallowing impairment affecting nutritional intake.

Dedicated interdisciplinary teams can join up with social initiatives and charities to provide holistic care and support the lifestyle factors to live better in older age.

Palliative and end of life care

Palliative and end of life care needs to remain an open topic with older people and not be one that is avoided or delayed given the unpredictable nature of dying in older age. Older people with communication difficulties will need support to be able to access these conversations and voice their opinions.

Provision of end of life care needs to be as well established amongst the older client group as it is with illness, such as cancer or other terminal illnesses. Of course, there is overlap between the two, with older people having a higher prevalence of terminal illness, but as mentioned in Chapter 9, older people tend to receive less quality palliative care in areas such as pain management.

Ahmed et al. (2021) make the case that 'dying well' as a frail older person includes minimising suffering, facilitating maintenance of independence for as long as possible and maintaining dignity when a person becomes more dependent on care. They report that palliative care for older people should include open communication with the older person and families, individualised and shared decision making, interdisciplinary team working and acceptance of flexibility and diversity to meet various needs of an older person at the end of their life.

Including older adults in service design and delivery

It is useful practice to get service feedback from clients and/or their families about their experiences of the service offered and to take any themes from this feedback to improve service delivery. Older adults may be less likely to make complaints about services or have difficulty accessing the methods to make a complaint if they are not confident with technology or have a communication impairment.

Methods of gaining feedback or making a complaint need to be accessible for older people so that their voices are heard.

In designing a service that will serve an older client group, it is the ideal that the opinions of potential clients themselves are included. This could include the layout of a clinic room or the appointment booking system or the methods of communication. In hospitals or care homes, they can give feedback on services, such as meal provision or activities on offer.

In doing this, older adults are more likely to be able to access the services offered and be able to get the best out of them.

Chapter summary

- The learning points from this book cover normal physiology of ageing, protective factors and rehabilitation, theory and clinical management of age-related communication and swallowing impairments, decision making and palliative care in older age.
- Communication and swallowing impairments in older age are part of a bigger picture that encompasses overall physical and cognitive fitness.

- In the future, healthcare services for older people need to include education on protective factors for significant ageing, screening of older people to identify those most at risk, early intervention and interdisciplinary team working, and good-quality, person-centred palliative care.

References

Ahmed, N, Ahmedzai, SH and Harwood, RH (2021) The Geriatrician's role in end of life care. *Age and Ageing*. 50: 366-369.

Maher, J et al. (2019) 268 can the swallow screening component of a frailty assessment be used to reliably direct clinical dysphagia assessment referrals? *Age and Ageing*. 48 (Suppl 3): iii17-iii65.

Travers, J et al. (2019) Delaying and reversing frailty: A systematic review of primary care interventions. *British Journal of General Practice*. 69 (678): e61-e69.

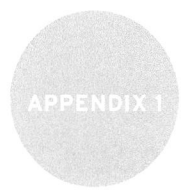

INTERNATIONAL DYSPHAGIA DIET STANDARDISATION INITIATIVE (IDDSI) FRAMEWORK

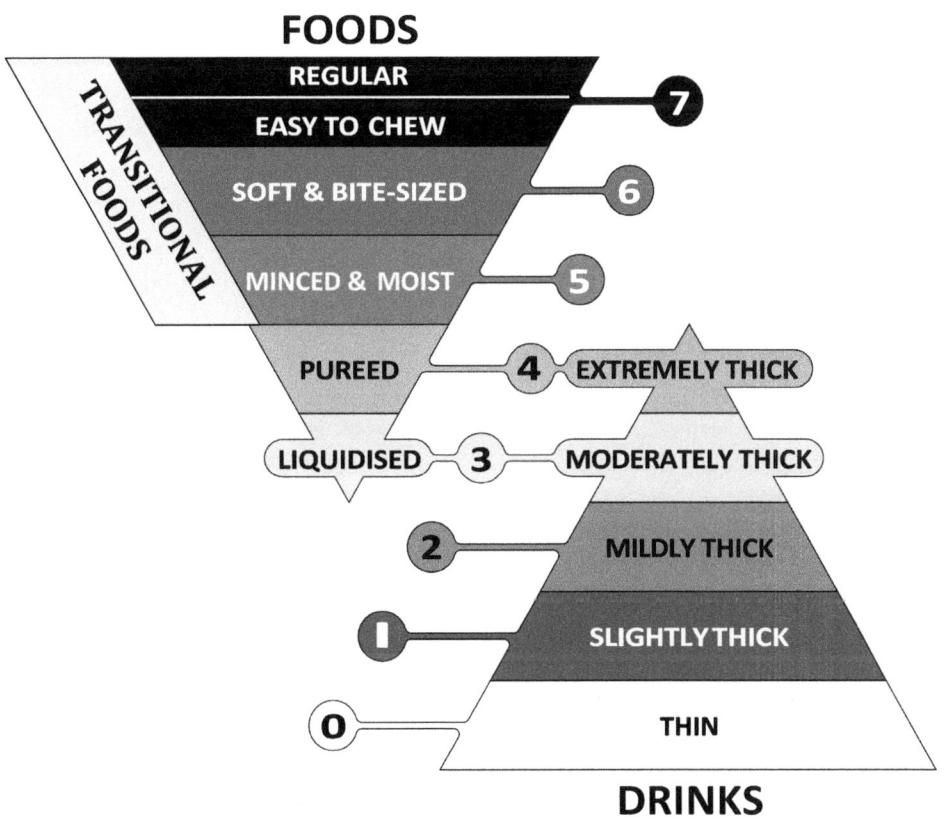

Index

Page locators in **bold** indicate a table. Page locators in *italics* indicate a diagram.